The Dr. Sebi Diet Cookbook with Pictures

The Nutritional Guide with Easy Alkaline Diet Recipes & Food List

21-Day Meal Plan Based on Dr. Sebi Products & Herbs

OLIVIA SHIELDS

DEDICATION

This book is dedicated to the millions of adults who want to change their lives!

Copyright © 2020 Olivia Shields

All rights reserved.

No part of this book may be reproduced in any form or by any electronic or mechanical means, except in the case of a brief quotation embodied in articles or reviews, without written permission from its publisher.
ISBN: 9798566451749

DISCLAIMER

The material and recipes contained in this book are provided for informational purposes only. Please consult with a qualified healthcare provider before making any changes in your diet or lifestyle. The author does not assume any liability or responsibility to anyone for the use of all or any information contained in this book, with respect to any loss or damage caused or alleged to be caused directly or indirectly from the provided information.

All images are from stock.adobe.com.

CONTENTS

Introduction 7

The Dr. Sebi Diet 8
  What is the Dr. Sebi Diet? 8
  Rules & Food Principles 10
  Is It Safe? 11
  Why Are Hybrid Products Dangerous? 13
  Benefits & Downsides 16
  Dr. Sebi's Supplements 18
  Weight Loss & Reverse Disease 20

Dr. Sebi's Food List 22
  Approved Products 22
    Vegetable List 23
    Fruit List 24
    Grain List 25
    Spices and Seasonings 25
    Teas, Oil, Nuts, and Seeds 26
  Permitted Products 28

21-Day Meal Plan 29

Dr. Sebi Inspired Recipes 39
  Soups 39
    Mushroom Soup 40
    Veggie Soup 42
    Soursop Soup 44
    Spicy Tomato Bean Soup 46
    Creamy Cucumber Gazpacho 48
  Salads 49
    "Potato" Salad 50
    Zucchini-and-Squash Salad 52
    Fresh Salad 54
    Quick Mango Salsa 55
    Chickpea Salad 56
    Pickle Salad 57
    Sautéed Kale 58

Main Dishes 59
- Vegetarian Pizza 60
- Mushroom Gravy 62
- Egg Foo Yung 64
- Teff Patties 66
- Waffles & Veggie "Chicken" 68
- Mushroom Strips 70
- Spaghetti Squash 72
- Walnut Filling 73
- Zucchini Bacon 74
- Homemade Pasta 76
- Quiche 78
- Veggie Alfredo 80
- Butternut Squash Fries 82
- Vegetable Quinoa 84
- Zucchini Patties 86
- Mashed Burros 88
- Baked Beans 90
- Sausage Links 92

Sauces 94
- Orange-Ginger Sauce 95
- Spicy Tomato Sauce 96
- Hempseed Mayonnaise 98
- Tomato Pizza Sauce 99
- Cheese Sauce 100
- Garlic Sauce 102
- Salsa Verde 103
- White Queso Dip 104

Special Ingredients 106
- Homemade Walnut Milk 107
- Aquafaba 108
- Homemade Coconut Milk 110
- Homemade Tahini Butter 111
- Homemade Date Sugar 112
- Homemade Date Syrup 113
- Homemade Hempseed Milk 114

Snacks & Bread 115

Tortillas 116
Tortilla Chips 118
Herb Bread 120
Chickpea "Tofu" 121
Kale Chips 122
Desserts **123**
Banana Pie 124
Mango Cheesecake 126
Coconut Waffle 128
Applesauce 129
French Toast 130
Alkaline Porridge 132
Date Balls 133
Strawberry Jam 134
Pancakes 135
Spelt Cookies 136
Coconut Tahini Cookies 138
Teff Tahini Cookies 139
Strawberry Banana Ice Cream 140
Smoothies **142**
Soursop Smoothie 143
Healthy Smoothie 144
Limeade 146
Cucumber-Ginger Water 147
Strawberry Milkshake 148
Cactus Smoothie 149
Prickly Pear Juice 150
Ginger Tea 151
Banana Milkshake 152
Strawberry Limeade 153
Soursop Tea 154
Ginger Shot 155
Green Smoothie 156
Peach Strawberry Smoothie 157
Conclusion **158**

INTRODUCTION

Are you ready to change your life, improve overall health and, in addition, lose weight? Do you want to cleanse your liver, detox your body and skin, remove phlegm and mucus, and naturally prevent some diseases such as Herpes and Diabetes? You can do it by sticking to just ONE thing—the Dr. Sebi Diet!

You are holding in your hands my second book about the Dr. Sebi Diet. I even became more immersed in this topic and gathered additional useful information about rules, food principles, benefits and downsides, dangers of GMO products, weight loss, and reverse diseases— this is not even the whole list! It turned out to be a complete nutritional guide to Dr. Sebi Diet.

Moreover, I have prepared for you a NEW portion of delicious food—77 NEW Easy Dr. Sebi-inspired recipes. Most recipes are new, and they are not recipes from my last book! You can be sure that you will get even more variety in everyday food. But if you haven't bought my first book yet, you can always purchase it on Amazon and have in your arsenal about 140 recipes from two books.

Specifically, in the next sections, you will learn:
- What is the Dr. Sebi Alkaline Diet?
- Is it safe or not?
- What are the main rules and food principles?
- Which products are in the Dr. Sebi food list?
- Why are hybrid products so dangerous?
- Which supplements are necessary to take Green Food Plus, Sea Moss, Viento, and others?
- What are the benefits and downsides of the Dr. Sebi diet?
- Does the diet of Dr. Sebi help with diabetes or herpes?
- Does the Dr. Sebi diet cleanse the liver?
- How can you lose weight by sticking to it?

Are you ready for a big portion of only useful information? Then let's go!

THE DR. SEBI DIET

WHAT IS THE DR. SEBI DIET?

The Dr. Sebi Diet was developed by Alfredo Darrington Bowman, a self-taught herbalist who found excellent nutritional value in some foods. Despite his name, however, Dr. Sebi did not hold a Ph.D., nor was he a medical practitioner.

He claimed these plant-based meals could help people prevent diseases and serve as treatment plans for chronic medical conditions, such as diabetes.

This diet is composed of greens, fruits, vegetables, grains, and other plants that are intended to create alkaline conditions in the body.

Why Was the Diet Developed?

The Dr. Sebi diet is a plant-based diet that rejuvenates body cells by eliminating toxic waste by alkalizing the blood.

When designing this diet, Dr. Sebi had in mind those people that wish to prevent or cure disease and improve their general health without depending on Western medicine. According to him, diseases result from the buildup of mucus in a region of the body. For instance, mucus buildup in your lungs is pneumonia. Similarly, diabetes is excessive mucus in your pancreas.

The doctor argues that alkaline environments do not encourage the existence of a disease. Diseases will only attack if your body is too acidic. His diet promises the restoration of the body's alkaline state. Detoxification of your body is also guaranteed when you religiously follow his diet.

Furthermore, this diet induces cell rejuvenation and the elimination of toxic substances from the blood and body, promoting improved health and stronger resistance to illnesses.

What Does the Diet Consist Of?

The diet consists of approved fruits, vegetables, grains, seeds, herbs, nuts, and oils. The Dr. Sebi diet is a diet for vegans as it doesn't include animal products. For the body to self-heal, the diet has to be followed consistently throughout your life.

For an in-depth analysis of what constitutes this popular diet, we will look closer at the details in the subsequent sections. They will include the types of foods to eat, the benefits and drawbacks of the diet, its significance to weight loss, the supplements involved, and how it reverses medical illnesses.

RULES & FOOD PRINCIPLES

There are strict food rules that need to be followed to gain optimal results from Dr. Sebi's diet. You will have to make it a routine to adhere to the program for an indefinite amount of time. It is a lifelong endeavor. Bowman claimed that for the body to continually heal itself, you will have to eat the listed foods regularly.

There are eight major rules you should follow when on the Dr. Sebi diet. The standards focus mainly on avoiding ultra-processed foods, animal products, and taking proprietary supplements.

- **Rule 1:** Consume products only from Dr. Sebi's food list.
- **Rule 2:** Drink 3.8 liters of water daily.
- **Rule 3:** One hour before taking your medications, take the recommended supplements.
- **Rule 4:** Animal products (including meat, milk, eggs, etc.) are not permitted.
- **Rule 5:** Alcohol consumption is not allowed.
- **Rule 6:** Do not eat wheat products. You are only supposed to eat "natural growing grains" from the nutritional guide.
- **Rule 7:** Do not use a microwave as it would kill your food.
- **Rule 8:** Avoid seedless or canned fruits.

From the description above, you can notice that Dr. Sebi's diet isn't rich in proteins because it prohibits lentils, some beans, soy, and animal products. Proteins are essential diet constituents as they are responsible for healthy joints, skin, and muscles.

You are required to buy Dr. Sebi's supplements to nourish your body cells and cleanse the body. There is a package that comes with 20 products for this function, although you can order a supplement according to your health problems.

Bio Ferro capsules, for instance, claim to cleanse one's blood, treat liver problems, boost the body's immunity, assist in weight loss, and solve digestive issues. Furthermore, the list of nutrients and their quantities is incomplete. Because of this, you won't know if your needs will be met.

IS IT SAFE?

Before embarking on this diet, you should first consult your physician. Avoid getting on the Dr. Sebi diet if you think you have kidney issues as it could just worsen your situation.

List of Alkaline-creating vegetables:
- Wheatgrass
- Barley grass
- Cauliflower
- Cabbage
- Broccoli
- Beets
- Eggplant
- Onion
- Garlic
- Lettuce
- Chlorella
- Mushrooms
- Green peas
- Zucchinis
- Beans
- Sweet potato
- Watercress
- Tomatoes
- Cucumber
- Celery
- Spinach
- Pumpkin
- Pepper.

List of Acid-creating products:
- Prunes
- Plums
- Beans
- Legumes

- Winter squash
- Olives
- Lentils
- Corn
- Blueberries
- Cranberries
- Coated and canned organic products.

Knowing the role of these nourishments assists in adjusting your body's inward pH.

WHY ARE HYBRID PRODUCTS DANGEROUS?

Crossbreeding and hybridization help come up with better animal and plant species. How is it beneficial?

Benefits of Hybridizing

First, the new species of plants will give produce that has better taste, thinner skin, or bigger size. Second, hybridized species tend to be more disease-resistant. They can resist drought and frost as well. Third, the developed species of animals prove more comfortable to manage or breed. They also give more meat, wool, and milk.

Drawbacks of Hybridizing

The developed species can negatively affect the environment. For instance, compared to their native counterparts, they may require more food and water. Also, they may be nutrient-hungry, thus depleting the minerals from the soil. This way, it is impossible for anything to grow on it. Another disadvantage of crossbreeding is that the new species may replace the native ones, which have proven to benefit local wildlife.

Since the life of a vegetable or fruit lies in its seed, you can identify a hybridized seed by looking at its seed. If the seed is absent, then the species is hybridized. However, several hybridized seeds contain seeds, for example, tomatoes.

Why Did Dr. Sebi Discourage Hybrid Foods?

In one of the eight rules of the Dr. Sebi diet, he advises against consuming hybrid foods. He based his reasons on their lack of life and high starch and sugar content. Furthermore, they do not have an ideal balance in minerals of the native species. In simple terms, a diet comprised of hybrid foods is a mineral-deficient diet.

Hybrid fruits taste better than the indigenous ones because of the higher sugar content, which isn't good for your pancreas. Also, compared to native species, hybrid fruits have a lower nutrient content. So, even though many of these fruits containing seeds, avoiding consuming seedless fruits is one of the easiest ways of preventing unnatural foods in your diet.

The Mucous Membrane

Several factors can compromise the body's immune system. One of them is nutrient-deficiency and acidic foods. With time, an inappropriate diet destroys the mucous membrane, paving the way for several health problems.

The mucous membrane is a lining that runs through your digestive, reproductive, and respiratory organs. It serves to prevent pathogens from entering our internal organs. It also prevents your body tissues from being dehydrated. Your vulnerability to disease increases if the membrane becomes very thin or gets broken.

For instance, a Helicobacter pylori infection may cause thinning or damage to the stomach's mucous membrane. Consequently, food will be broken down by hydrochloric acid in the stomach, and you may develop ulcers or gastritis.

What Causes Damage to the Mucous Membrane?

It could result from many things, such as its location. Here are the common causes:
- Acidic food
- Dehydration resulting from alcohol
- Drug abuse or tobacco use
- Poor hygiene practices
- Stress
- Chemotherapy
- Mouth breathing
- Radiation therapy
- Depression
- Malnutrition
- Infection
- Immunosuppression.

The bottom line is that hybrid foods aren't unhealthy, and they are not dangerous to eat, but they are unnatural in the sense that man created them.

Is It Safe to Eat Hybridized Foods?

Most of the foods we eat today have at some point been tampered with by man. It isn't easy to avoid them, but it can be done. That is why the foods recommended by Dr. Sebi are of limited variety. Followers of this diet would deprive themselves of many essential nutrients if they followed it without taking the recommended herbal remedies and supplements.

Most diets today consist of acidic foods. For balancing PH levels, avoid acidic foods. Instead, eat more alkaline foods.

BENEFITS & DOWNSIDES

The Dr. Sebi diet comes with its benefits and drawbacks too.

The Diet's Benefits

Here are some of its benefits:
- It promotes the consumption of several fruits and vegetables rich in vitamins, fiber, plant compounds, and minerals.
- The diet consists of plant compounds that boost the body's immunity and combat inflammation.
- The program aids in weight loss. According to a recent study, a diet of vegetables yielded better weight loss results than other eating regimens that are less prohibitive. Participants in the study lost 7.5% of their total body weight after being on a vegetable diet for six months.
- It aids in controlling craving. A recently-concluded report in male youth found that they felt more fulfilled after eating dinner consisting of beans and peas than one consisting of meat.
- The diet helps in changing microorganisms inside the gut. A recently concluded study showed that feeding on plant-based diets could modify and improve the gut microbiome, lowering the risk of ailments.
- Dr. Sebi's diet diminishes the danger of contracting a coronary illness. Feeding on this diet also reduces the risks of diabetes and metabolic disorders.
- Given the high fiber content in the diet consisting mainly of vegetables and whole grains, you will be able to handle constipation better and ease your bowel movements.

The Diet's Downsides

Despite all the above-listed benefits, the diet has its drawbacks:
- **Highly Restrictive**

It is one of the major drawbacks of Dr. Sebi's diet. Many food groups are restricted by this diet—for example, animal products, beans, lentil wheat, and some fruits and vegetables.

How strict is the program? Only certain fruits can be consumed. For instance, you can eat plum or cherry tomatoes but not roma tomatoes.

Following such a rigid diet can be torturous. It can negatively affect your relationship with food, as it prohibits many foods. The diet can make you develop harmful behaviors, like achieving fullness by using supplements.

- **Lacks in Proteins and Other Vital Nutrients**

The foods recommended by Dr. Sebi are excellent nutrition sources. The protein content of the diet, however, raises many questions. The foods are not good protein sources. This is unfortunate given the role of proteins in skin structure, enzyme production, and muscle growth.

To satisfy your protein needs, you will have to consume large volumes of the listed foods. The foods listed by Dr. Sebi are rich in beta carotene, vitamins C and E, and Potassium. They, however, have low calcium, omega-3, iron, vitamin B12, and D content.

- **Not Science-Based**

There is no scientific evidence to support claims that Dr. Sebi's diet can cure some illnesses. The doctor claims that the supplements and foods in his plant-based diet control the production of acid in the body. However, your body makes sure there is a balance between acids and bases to keep the blood pH between 7.36 & 7.44. It naturally alkalizes your body.

- **Unsustainability**

Processed foods are not welcome in Dr. Sebi's diet. The foods approved by Dr. Sebi may prove hard to find in restaurants and average supermarkets. You may find it difficult to prepare them at home, thus lowering your chances of sticking with the diet.

DR. SEBI'S SUPPLEMENTS

In addition to eating the foods listed in Dr. Sebi's nutritional guide, you will also be required to buy his proprietary supplements. Bowman guaranteed they would aid in cleansing your body and nourishing your cells.

The recommended package is the all-inclusive option, consisting of all 20 of the available supplements. This is said to be the best option because it is the fastest means of cleansing and restoring the body.

Alternatively, you can opt to purchase individual supplements based on your health goals. For more details, let's take a look at some of the supplements and what they offer:

- **Sea Moss/Seaweed** – This nutritious plant is a rich source of calcium, magnesium, iron, and ninety-two other essential minerals. It also contains many vitamins and is quite versatile in how you can ingest it. Sea moss can be incorporated in baking, blended into smoothies, used as an ingredient for gravies, ice creams, and fashioned into desserts. It is well known for its healing aspects and ability to promote a balanced restoration of the mucous membrane, thus improving your overall health. The ailments it can help treat include skin conditions.
- **Uterine Wash and Oil** – It is used in cleansing and restoring the natural state of your vaginal canal. Pour boiling water (8 oz) over one tablespoon of the herb, wait for it to cool, and use it to douche.
- **Viento** – This is an energizer and cleanser. It will revitalize your body and increase the oxygen levels in your brain and blood. It is rich in iron, which is used in the formation of hemoglobin in red blood cells. The supplement also works on your kidneys and the lymphatic, respiratory, and central nervous systems. Take a daily dosage of four capsules.
- **Tooth Powder** – This unique herb combination helps cleanse your teeth. Apart from that, it nourishes gums and

retards gum disease and tooth decay. After wetting the brush, add about 1/8 of the powder then brush.
- **Testo** – By nourishing your endocrine system, this supplement aids in the balance of hormones. It increases virility and betters sexual responsiveness. Additionally, Testo encourages a healthy flow of blood to male genitalia.
- **Green Food Plus** – This formula contains several minerals. It consists of herbs rich in chlorophyll for the whole body. Apart from promoting nourishment and good health, this supplement also helps the heart, the central nervous system, and the brain. Take four capsules daily.
- **Banju** – Conditions of the central nervous system—such as irritability, stress, insomnia, and irritability—can be addressed with this supplement. It was made for kids with ADD and ADHD but is also effective in mature people. The dosage is two tablespoons twice a day.
- **Iron Plus** – This offers iron-rich nourishment to the brain, blood, and central nervous system. It was developed to purify and provide strength to your entire body. This supplement also prevents inflammation. The dosage is two tablespoons per day.
- **Hair Food Oil** – It provides nourishment to the scalp and hair. For best results, apply daily.
- **Hair Follicle Fortifier** – Its role is cleansing and strengthening hair follicles to promote the growth of new hair.
- **Bio Ferro Capsules** – They purify and nourish your blood, and contain herbs rich in iron phosphate and several other minerals that nourish and strengthen your entire system.

It is worth noting that these supplements do not provide a guide on all the nutrients in them and in what quantities. Contact your doctor to discuss this further.

WEIGHT LOSS & REVERSE DISEASE

Is the Dr. Sebi Diet Effective for Weight Loss?

Although it wasn't originally made for this purpose, following it can help you lose weight. It discourages Western diets that consist mainly of ultra-processed food loaded with sugar, salt, and fat. Instead, it is plant-based, and people that follow it tend to have lower heart disease and obesity rates than those that follow the Western diet.

A one-year study was done on 65 people. It was found that those who strictly followed the whole-food and low-fat diet lost more weight than those that didn't. After six months, those who adhered to this diet had gotten rid of 26 pounds while the others lost three pounds.

Furthermore, most of the recommended foods have low-calorie content except for seeds, nuts, oils, and avocados. Therefore, eating large portions of the approved foods won't result in surplus calories. Sadly, most people regain their lost weight as soon as they resume their regular diet.

Does It Help to Reverse Diseases?

The question of whether Dr. Sebi's diet can reverse diseases is one that still sparks debate today. Alfredo Bowman championed his cause that the diet could provide relief to people with various ailments. Among others, these include diabetes, heart conditions, liver problems, herpes, and kidney issues.

His premise suggested that the foods altered your body's pH and made it more alkaline, thus aiding in fighting disease. Science, however, says otherwise. According to research, foods can alter your urine's alkalinity level, but they do not affect the blood's pH.

However, this does not mean that all is lost. On the contrary, this diet has many health and medical benefits.

Fruits and vegetables improve heart function and strengthen it. It makes the heart capable of combating disease and reduces the risk of heart attacks.

Because the diet is low in fat, it also serves as an excellent way to prevent atherosclerosis and the accumulation of fatty deposits in your blood vessels. Healthy blood vessels allow proper blood flow and minimize strain on your heart.

Your body will also get a healthy balance of macronutrients and vitamins from the listed foods. It fosters an overall improvement in health.

Since this diet is rich in fiber, it can help people suffering from constipation cope with the condition and even reverse it. Seeds, vegetables, fruits, and nuts all play critical roles in easing bowel movements.

Dr. Sebi's diet has many health benefits, but it comes with several drawbacks. Fortunately, there is a way around them. By consuming plant-based protein sources such as beans and lentils, you can meet the nutritional needs of a well-rounded diet and gain the most benefit. If you suffer from any chronic condition or you are taking certain medications, consult your doctor before transitioning to this diet.

DR. SEBI'S FOOD LIST
APPROVED PRODUCTS

Dr. Sebi strongly believed that people should strictly eat only non-GMO foods. This approved list of products includes vegetables and fruits which are not seedless or otherwise altered, and they contain many minerals and vitamins that occur naturally.

GMO foods are those that result from unnatural cross-pollination. Dr. Sebi strongly advocated against these foods because they change the electrical composition, genetic structure, and pH balance to its detriment. This is the reason why his list of foods consists only of those that are unaltered and contain many naturally-occurring vitamins and minerals.

While the vegetable list is extensive, the list of fruits is much smaller since many types of fruits should be avoided, according to Dr. Sebi. The herbs list is the shortest because it is difficult to find herbs that have remained unaltered.

However, in its entirety, this prepared Dr. Sebi Food List is long and diverse. It contains a variety of options to create a wide array of delicious dishes.

As promised, I want to provide you with **a shopping list of approved Doctor Sebi products for FREE.** It will help to prevent you from buying unnecessary products. This file will be sent to your email in PDF format and can be opened on your phone, tablet or laptop.

Just follow this link or scan QR Code to sign up and receive your shopping list!

http://bit.ly/drsebi-2

VEGETABLE LIST

Vegetables	
Amaranth Greens (Callaloo, a variety of greens)	Wild Arugula
Avocado	Bell Peppers
Chayote (Mexican Squash)	Cucumber
Dandelion Greens	Garbanzo Beans
Izote (Cactus flower, Cactus leaf)	Kale
Lettuce (all types, except Iceberg)	Mushrooms (all types, except Shitake)
Nopales (Mexican Cactus)	Okra
Olives	Onions
Sea Vegetables (Wakame, Arame, Hijiki, Dulse, Nori)	Squash
Tomato (Cherry and Plum only)	Tomatillo
Turnip Greens	Zucchini
Watercress	Purslane (Verdolaga)

FRUIT LIST

Fruits	
Apples	Bananas (Baby or Burro only)
Berries (all, except Cranberries)	Cantaloupe
Cherries	Currants
Dates	Figs
Grapes (seeded only)	Limes (Key Limes preferred, with seeds)
Mango	Melons (seeded only)
Orange (Seville or sour preferred)	Papayas
Peaches	Pears
Plums	Prickly Pear (Cactus Fruit)
Prunes	Raisins (seeded only)
Soft Jelly Coconuts	Soursop (West Indian or Latin markets)
Tamarind	

GRAIN LIST

Grains	
Amaranth	Fonio
Kamut	Quinoa
Rye	Spelt
Tef	Wild Rice

SPICES AND SEASONINGS

Mild Flavors	
Basil	Bay Leaf
Cloves	Dill
Oregano	Savory
Sweet Basil	Tarragon
Thyme	

Sweet Flavors	
Pure Agave Syrup (from cactus)	Date Sugar

Pungent & Spice Flavors	
Achiote	Cayenne Pepper
African Bird Pepper	Onion Powder
Habanero	Sage

Salty Flavors	
Pure Sea Salt	Powdered Granulated Seaweed (Kelp, Dulce, Nori – have a "sea taste")

Sweet Flavors	
Pure Agave Syrup (from cactus)	Date Sugar

TEAS, OIL, NUTS, AND SEEDS

Herbal Teas	
Burdock	Chamomile
Elderberry	Fennel
Ginger	Raspberry
Tila	

Oils

Olive Oil (Do not cook)	Coconut Oil (Do not cook)
Grape Seed Oil	Hempseed Oil
Avocado Oil	Sesame Oil

Nuts & Seeds

Hemp seeds	Raw Sesame Seeds
Raw Sesame "Tahini" Butter	Walnuts
Brazil Nuts	

PERMITTED PRODUCTS

Any products that are not from the approved Dr. Sebi list of food are not permitted:
- Seedless fruits
- Wheat
- Dairy
- Processed foods
- Soy products
- Eggs
- Red meat
- Poultry
- Fish
- Canned vegetables or fruits
- Sugar (except agave syrup and date sugar)
- Fortified foods
- Foods made with baking powder
- Yeast
- Restaurant or takeout foods
- Alcohol.

Remember: According to the Dr. Sebi diet, many vegetables, grains, fruits, nuts, seeds, and oils are not allowed! Only products from the approved food list can be eaten.

21-DAY MEAL PLAN

Before checking the 21-Day Meal Plan, please read the useful rules that I have prepared for you. It will help to save time during cooking! :)

Rules:
1. Carefully read everyday tips (example – Tips for Day 1) BEFORE you start preparing any meal.
2. Save your time for your family, friends, etc. Don't spend too much time in the kitchen! Make more portions, freeze them, or store in the fridge. You'll see how to do this in everyday tips and at the bottom of recipes.
3. You don't have to eat snacks if you are not hungry—only if you have the desire.
4. If you want, you can add extras to your meal—salads from fresh greens and vegetables, sauces, fruits, pure agave syrup, tortillas, etc.

Day 1
- Breakfast – Coconut Waffle *(on page 128)* with agave syrup and fruits
- Lunch - Mushroom Soup[1] *(on page 40)* with Herb Bread[2] *(on page 120)*
- Dinner - Zucchini-and-Squash Salad *(on page 52)*
- Snack – Soursop Smoothie *(on page 143)*

Tips for Day 1:
1. Store an extra portion of *Mushroom Soup* in a fridge for Day 2 (look at lunch).
2. Keep the leftover of *Herb Bread* for Day 2 (look at breakfast and lunch).

Day 2
- Breakfast – French Toast[1] *(on page 130)*
- Lunch - Mushroom Soup[1] *(on page 40)* with Herb Bread[1] *(on page 120)*

- Dinner - Quiche[2, 3, 4] *(on page 78)*
- Snack - Strawberry Milkshake *(on page 148)*

Tips for Day 2:
1. If you follow my everyday tips, you have already cooked *Mushroom Soup* and *Herb Bread*.
2. Store an extra portion of *Quiche* in a fridge for Day 3 (look at dinner).
3. Cook 2 more portion of *"Cheese" Sauce* for Day 3 (look at lunch and snack).
4. Make an extra batch of *"Garlic" Sauce* for Day 4 (look at lunch).

Day 3
- Breakfast – Alkaline Porridge *(on page 132)* with fruits
- Lunch - Veggie Alfredo[1, 2] *(on page 80)*
- Dinner - Quiche[1] *(on page 78)*
- Snack - Tortilla Chips[3] *(on page 118)* with "Cheese" Sauce[1] *(on page 100)*

Tips for Day 3:
1. If you follow my everyday tips, you have already cooked *Quiche* and *"Cheese" Sauce*.
2. Freeze 4 extra portions of *Homemade Pasta* for Day 5 (look at lunch), Day 8 (look at dinner), Day 17 (look at dinner), Day 21 (look at lunch).
3. Cook an extra batch of *Tortilla Chips* for Day 4 (look at snack).

Day 4
- Breakfast – Coconut Tahini Cookies[2] *(on page 138)*
- Lunch - Waffles & Veggie "Chicken"[3] *(on page 68)* with "Garlic" Sauce[1] *(on page 102)*
- Dinner - Vegetarian Pizza[4] *(on page 60)*
- Snack - Tortilla Chips[1] *(on page 118)* with Quick Mango Salsa *(on page 55)*

Tips for Day 4:
1. If you follow my everyday tips, you have already cooked *Tortilla Chips* and *"Garlic" Sauce*.
2. Cook an extra batch of *Coconut Tahini Cookies* for Day 5 (look at snack).
3. Cook an extra portion of *Veggie "Chicken"* for Day 5 (look at dinner).
4. Cook an extra portion of *Vegetarian Pizza* for Day 5 (look at breakfast).

Day 5
- Breakfast – Vegetarian Pizza[1] *(on page 60)*
- Lunch - Veggie Soup[1,2] *(on page 42)*
- Dinner - Spaghetti Squash[3] *(on page 72)* with Veggie "Chicken"[1] *(on page 68)*
- Snack - Coconut Tahini Cookies[1] *(on page 138)*

Tips for Day 5:
1. If you follow my everyday tips, you have already cooked *Vegetarian Pizza*, *Veggie "Chicken"*, *Coconut Tahini Cookies* and frozen *Homemade Pasta* for *Veggie Soup*.
2. Store an extra portion of *Veggie Soup* in a fridge for Day 6 (look at lunch).
3. Make and extra portion of *Spaghetti Squash* for Day 6 (look at dinner).

Day 6
- Breakfast – Banana Pie[2] *(on page 124)*
- Lunch - Veggie Soup[1] *(on page 42)*
- Dinner - Egg Foo Yung[1] *(on page 64)* with Mushroom Gravy[3] *(on page 62)*
- Snack - Cactus Smoothie *(on page 149)*

Tips for Day 6:
1. If you follow my everyday tips, you have already cooked *Spaghetti Squash* and *Veggie Soup*.

2. Store an extra portion of *Banana Pie* in a fridge for Day 7 (look at breakfast).
3. Make an extra portion of *Mushroom Gravy* for Day 7 (look at dinner).

Day 7
- Breakfast – Banana Pie[1] *(on page 124)*
- Lunch - Egg Foo Yung[1] *(on page 64)* with Orange-Ginger Sauce[2] *(on page 95)*
- Dinner - Mashed Burros *(on page 88)* with Mushroom Gravy[1] *(on page 62)*
- Snack - Spelt Cookies[3] *(on page 136)*

Tips for Day 7:
1. If you follow my everyday tips, you have already cooked *Banana Pie, Egg Goo Yung* and *Mushroom Gravy*.
2. Make an extra portion of *Orange-Ginger Sauce* for Day 8 (look at dinner).
3. Keep an extra batch of *Spelt Cookies* for Day 8 (look at breakfast).

Day 8
- Breakfast – Spelt Cookies[1] *(on page 136)*
- Lunch - Soursop Soup[2] *(on page 44)*
- Dinner - Teff Patties *(on page 66)* with Orange-Ginger Sauce[1] *(on page 95)* and cooked Homemade Pasta[1] *(on page 76)*
- Snack - Prickly Pear Juice *(on page 150)*

Tips for Day 8:
1. If you follow my everyday tips, you have already cooked *Spelt Cookies, Orange-Ginger Sauce* and frozen *Homemade Pasta*.
2. Store an extra portion of *Soursop Soup* in a fridge for Day 9 (look at lunch).

Day 9
- Breakfast – Pancakes *(on page 135)* with Strawberry Jam[2] *(on page 134)*
- Lunch - Soursop Soup[1] *(on page 44)*
- Dinner - Chickpea Salad[3] *(on page 56)*
- Snack – Kale Chips[4] *(on page 122)* with Salsa Verde[5] *(on page 103)*

Tips for Day 9:
1. If you follow my everyday tips, you have already cooked *Soursop Soup.*
2. Store an extra batch of *Strawberry Jam* for Day 10 (look at breakfast).
3. Keep an extra portion of *Hempseed Mayonnaise* for Day 10 (look at lunch).
4. Make an extra batch of *Kale Chips* for Day 10 (look at snack)
5. Make an extra portion of *Salsa Verde* for Day 10 (look at snack).

Day 10
- Breakfast – cooked porridge with Strawberry Jam[1] *(on page 134)*
- Lunch - Zucchini Bacon[2] *(on page 74)* with Hempseed Mayonnaise[1] *(on page 98)* and cooked wild rice
- Dinner – Baked Beans[3] *(on page 90)* with Tortillas *(on page 116)*
- Snack - Kale Chips[1] *(on page 122)* with Salsa Verde[1] *(on page 103)*

Tips for Day 10:
1. If you follow my everyday tips, you have already cooked *Strawberry Jam, Hempseed Mayonnaise, Kale Chips* and *Salsa Verde.*
2. Make an extra portion of *Zucchini Bacon* for Day 11 (look at dinner).

3. Cook an extra portion of *Baked Beans* for Day 11 (look at lunch).

Day 11
- Breakfast – <u>Mango Cheesecake</u>[2] *(on page 126)*
- Lunch – <u>Baked Beans</u>[1] *(on page 90)* with cooked kamut
- Dinner - <u>Zucchini Bacon</u>[1] *(on page 74)* and <u>Fresh Salad</u> *(on page 54)*
- Snack - <u>Teff Tahini Cookies</u>[3] *(on page 139)*

Tips for Day 11:
1. If you follow my everyday tips, you have already cooked *Baked Beans* and *Zucchini Bacon*.
2. Store the leftover of *Mango Cheesecake* for Day 12 (look at breakfast).
3. Make an extra portion of *Teff Tahini Cookies* for Day 12 (look at snack).

Day 12
- Breakfast – <u>Mango Cheesecake</u>[1] *(on page 126)*
- Lunch – <u>Vegetable Quinoa</u>[2] *(on page 84)*
- Dinner – <u>Butternut Squash Fries</u> *(on page 82)* with salad
- Snack - <u>Teff Tahini Cookies</u>[1] *(on page 139)*

Tips for Day 12:
1. If you follow my everyday tips, you have already cooked *Mango Cheesecake* and *Teff Tahini Cookies*.
2. Keep an extra portion of *Vegetable Quinoa* for Day 13 (look at lunch).

Day 13
- Breakfast – <u>Banana Pie</u>[2] *(on page 124)*
- Lunch - <u>Vegetable Quinoa</u>[1] *(on page 84)*
- Dinner - <u>Zucchini Patties</u>[3] *(on page 86)* with salad
- Snack – <u>Date Balls</u>[4] *(on page 133)*

Tips for Day 13:
1. If you follow my everyday tips, you have already cooked *Vegetable Quinoa*.
2. Keep the leftover of *Banana Pie* in a fridge for Day 14 (look at breakfast).
3. Make an extra portion of *Zucchini Patties* for Day 14 (look at lunch).
4. Cook an extra portion of *Date Balls* for Day 14 (look at snack).

Day 14
- Breakfast – Banana Pie[1] *(on page 124)*
- Lunch - Zucchini Patties[1] *(on page 86)* with cooked amaranth
- Dinner – "Potato" Salad[2] *(on page 50)*
- Snack – Date Balls[1] *(on page 133)*

Tips for Day 14:
1. If you follow my everyday tips, you have already cooked *Banana Pie, Zucchini Patties* and *Date Balls*.
2. Cook an extra portion of *"Potato" Salad* for Day 15 (look at dinner).

Day 15
- Breakfast – cooked teff with Applesauce[2] *(on page 129)*
- Lunch - Spicy Tomato Bean Soup[3] *(on page 46)* with Herb Bread[4] *(on page 120)*
- Dinner - "Potato" Salad[1] *(on page 50)*
- Snack – Banana Milkshake *(on page 152)*

Tips for Day 15:
1. If you follow my everyday tips, you have already cooked *"Potato" Salad*.
2. Make an extra portion of *Applesauce* for Day 16 (look at breakfast).
3. Keep the leftover of *Spicy Tomato Bean Soup* for Day 16 (look at lunch).

4. Keep the leftover of *Herb Bread* for Day 16 (look at breakfast and lunch).

Day 16
- Breakfast – <u>French Toast</u>[1] *(on page 130)* with <u>Applesauce</u>[1] *(on page 129)*
- Lunch – <u>Spicy Tomato Bean Soup</u>[1] *(on page 46)* with <u>Herb Bread</u>[1] *(on page 120)*
- Dinner – <u>Sausage Links</u>[2] *(on page 92)* with <u>Fresh Salad</u> *(on page 54)*
- Snack – <u>Green Smoothie</u> *(on page 156)*

Tips for Day 16:
1. If you follow my everyday tips, you have already cooked *Applesauce, Spicy Tomato Bean Soup* and *Herb Bread* for *French Toast.*
2. Cook more *Sausage Links* for Day 17 (look at lunch).

Day 17
- Breakfast – <u>Coconut Waffle</u> *(on page 128)* with agave syrup and fruits
- Lunch – <u>Sausage Links</u>[1] *(on page 92)* with cooked fonio.
- Dinner – cooked <u>Homemade Pasta</u>[1] *(on page 76)* with <u>Walnut Filling</u>[2] *(on page 73)*
- Snack – <u>Peach Strawberry Smoothie</u> *(on page 157)*

Tips for Day 17:
1. If you follow my everyday tips, you have already cooked *Sausage Links* and cooked *Homemade Pasta.*
2. Keep the leftover of *Walnut Filling* for Day 18 (look at lunch).

Day 18
- Breakfast – <u>Pancakes</u> *(on page 135)* with <u>Applesauce</u>[2] *(on page 129)*
- Lunch - <u>Walnut Filling</u>[1] *(on page 73)* with cooked spelt

- Dinner – Mushroom Strips[3] *(on page 70)* with Tomato Pizza Sauce[3] *(on page 99)* and salad
- Snack – Healthy Smoothie *(on page 144)*

Tips for Day 18:
1. If you follow my everyday tips, you have already cooked *Walnut Filling*.
2. Make an extra batch of *Applesauce* for Day 19 (look at breakfast).
3. Make an extra portion of *Mushroom Strips* and *Tomato Pizza Sauce* for Day 19 (look at snack).

Day 19
- Breakfast – cooked porridge with Applesauce[1] *(on page 129)*
- Lunch - Creamy Cucumber Gazpacho[2] *(on page 48)* with Chickpea "Tofu"[3] *(on page 121)*
- Dinner – Quiche[4] *(on page 78)*
- Snack – Mushroom Strips[1] *(on page 70)* with Tomato Pizza Sauce[1] *(on page 99)*

Tips for Day 19:
1. If you follow my everyday tips, you have already cooked *Applesauce, Mushroom Strips* and *Tomato Pizza Sauce*.
2. Keep the leftover of *Creamy Cucumber Gazpacho* for Day 20 (look at lunch).
3. Make an extra portion of *Chickpea "Tofu"* for Day 20 (look at snack).
4. Keep the leftover of *Quiche* for Day 20 (look at breakfast).

Day 20
- Breakfast – Quiche[1] *(on page 78)*
- Lunch - Creamy Cucumber Gazpacho[1] *(on page 48)* with Tortillas *(on page 116)*
- Dinner – Baked Beans[2] *(on page 90)* with Tortillas *(on page 116)*

- Snack – <u>Chickpea "Tofu"</u>[1] *(on page 121)* with <u>Tortillas</u> *(on page 116)*

Tips for Day 20:
1. If you follow my everyday tips, you have already cooked *Quiche, Creamy Cucumber Gazpacho* and *Chickpea "Tofu"*.
2. Cook and extra portion of *Baked Beans* for Day 21 (look at dinner).

Day 21
- Breakfast – <u>Spelt Cookies</u> *(on page 136)*
- Lunch - <u>Veggie Alfredo</u>[1] *(on page 80)*
- Dinner – <u>Baked Beans</u>[1] *(on page 90)* with <u>Pickle Salad</u> *(on page 57)*
- Snack – <u>Strawberry Banana Ice Cream</u> *(on page 140)*

Tips for Day 21:
1. If you follow my everyday tips, you have already cooked *Baked Beans* and frozen *Homemade Pasta*.

DR. SEBI INSPIRED RECIPES
SOUPS

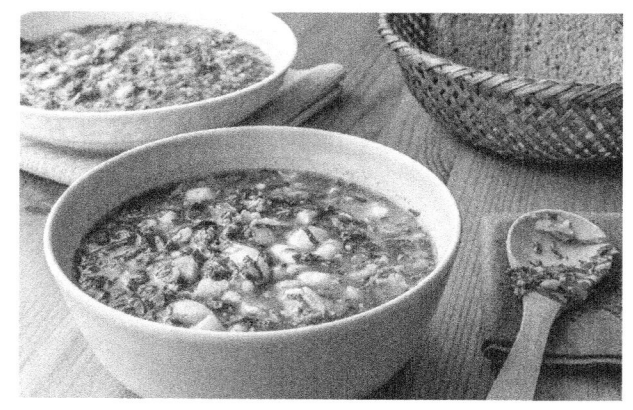

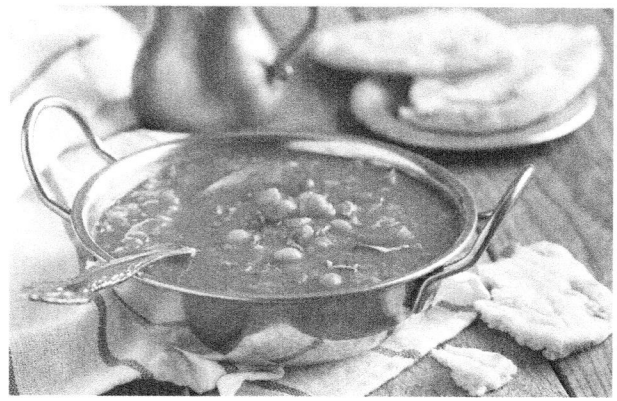

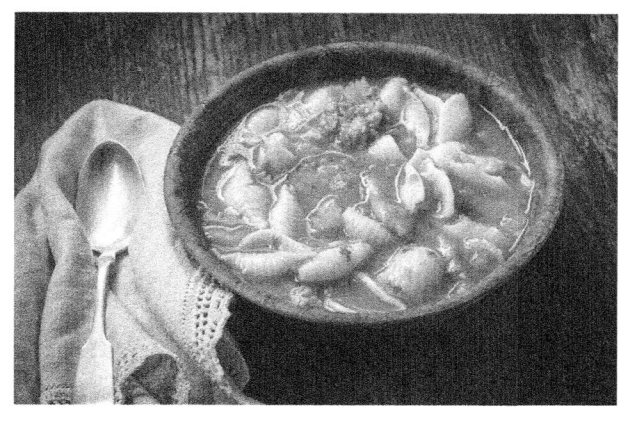

MUSHROOM SOUP

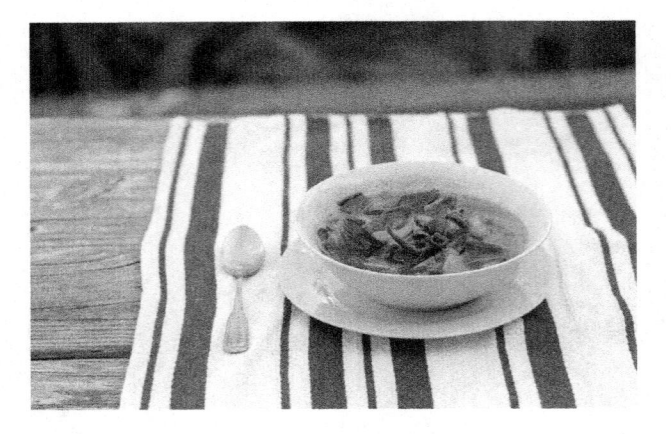

Cooking Time: 3 Hours 20 Minutes
Serving Size: 4–6 Servings

Ingredients

- 3 cups of chopped Portabella Mushrooms
- 1 cup of cooked Garbanzo Beans
- 2 cups of *Aquafaba (see recipe on page 108)*
- 1 cup of chopped Kale
- 2 diced Plum Tomatoes
- 1 cup of diced White Onions
- 1/2 cup of diced Green Bell Peppers
- 1/2 cup of diced Red Bell Peppers
- 1/2 cup of diced Butternut Squash
- 1/2 cup of chopped Red Onions
- 2 teaspoons of Pure Sea Salt
- 2 teaspoons of Onion Powder
- 1 teaspoon of Basil
- 1 teaspoon of Sage
- 1 teaspoon of Savory
- 1 teaspoon of Oregano
- 1/2 teaspoon of Ginger Powder
- 1/2 teaspoon of Thyme

- 1/4 teaspoon of Cayenne Powder**
- 2 tablespoons of Grapeseed Oil
- 2 cups of Spring Water

Cooking Instructions
1. Prepare all ingredients and put them in a slow cooker. Mix them well.
2. Cook soup on high heat for 3 hours. Stir occasionally.
3. If you don't have a slow cooker, you can cook it on a stovetop. Put all ingredients in a large pot, bring to a boil, reduce to low heat, and simmer for an hour. Stir occasionally.
4. Serve*** and enjoy your Mushroom Soup!

Useful Tips

* If you don't have prepared *Aquafaba*, add an extra 4 cups of Spring Water instead.

** If you don't like spicy soup, you can omit Cayenne Powder.

*** You can serve Mushroom Soup with our *Tortillas (see recipe on page 116)* or *Herb Bread (see recipe on page 120)*.

VEGGIE SOUP

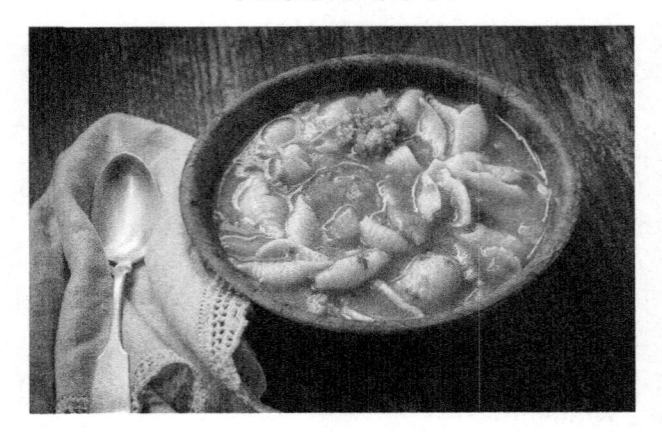

Cooking Time: 1 Hour 20 Minutes
Serving Size: 12 Servings

Ingredients
- 4 cups of cooked Garbanzo Beans
- 2–4 cups of *Homemade Pasta (see recipe on page 76)*
- 4 cups of chopped Mushrooms
- 1 cup of Quinoa (optional)
- 3 diced Plum Tomatoes
- 1 chopped Yellow Squash
- 1 chopped Zucchini Squash
- 2 cups of chopped Butternut Squash
- 1 cup of chopped Red Bell Peppers
- 1 cup of chopped Green Bell Peppers
- 1 chopped Red Onion
- 2 tablespoons of Pure Sea Salt
- 2 tablespoons of Grapeseed Oil
- 2 teaspoons of Basil
- 2 teaspoons of Oregano
- 1 teaspoon of Dill
- 1–2 teaspoons of Cayenne Powder
- 1 gallon of Spring Water

Cooking Instructions
1. In a large pot, pour Spring Water into it, and put on high heat.
2. Prepare all vegetables (chop or dice them).
3. Put all ingredients (except *Homemade Pasta*) and seasonings in the pot. Bring to a boil, reduce to low heat, and simmer for about 1 hour.
4. Stir every 12–15 minutes.
5. Add *Homemade Pasta* 5 minutes before it's cooked.
6. Serve* and enjoy your Veggie Soup!

Useful Tips
* You can serve Veggie Soup with our *Tortillas (see recipe on page 116)* or *Herb Bread (see recipe on page 120)*.

SOURSOP SOUP

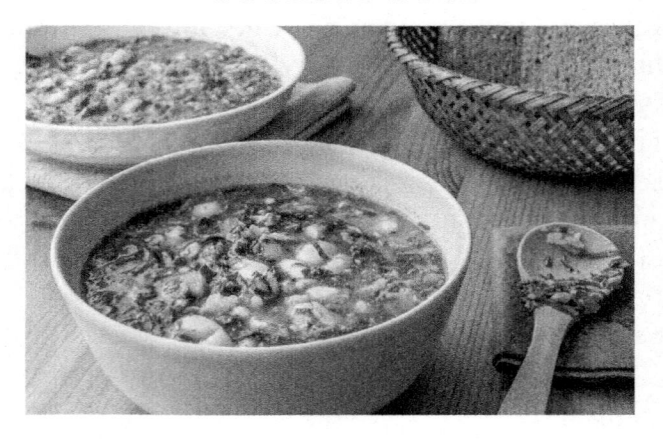

Cooking Time: 1 Hour 20 Minutes
Serving Size: 6–8 Servings

Ingredients

- 4–6 Soursop Leaves
- 2 cups of chopped Kale
- 1 diced Chayote Squash
- 1 cup of Quinoa*
- 1 cup of chopped Red Bell Peppers
- 1 cup of chopped Green Bell Peppers
- 1 cup of chopped Onions
- 1 cup of diced Zucchini
- 1 cup of diced Summer Squash
- 3 tablespoons of Onion Powder
- 4 teaspoons of Pure Sea Salt
- 1 tablespoon of minced Ginger
- 1 tablespoon of Oregano
- 1 tablespoon of Basil
- 1/4 teaspoon of Cayenne Powder**
- 12–16 cups of Spring Water

Cooking Instructions
1. Rinse the Soursop Leaves, put them in a large pot, and pour in 4 cups of Spring Water.
2. Boil leaves for 15–20 minutes.
3. Take the leaves out of the broth.
4. Prepare all vegetables (chop or dice them).
5. Put all ingredients* and seasonings** in the pot. Pour in 8 cups of Spring Water.
6. Bring to a boil, reduce to medium heat, and cook for 30–40 minutes.
7. Stir every 12–15 minutes.
8. Serve*** and enjoy your Soursop Soup!

Useful Tips
* If you don't have/like Quinoa, add Wild Rice or *Homemade Pasta (see recipe on page 76)* instead.
** If you don't like spicy soup, you can omit Cayenne Powder.
*** You can serve Soursop Soup with our *Tortillas (see recipe on page 116)* or *Herb Bread (see recipe on page 120)*.

SPICY TOMATO BEAN SOUP

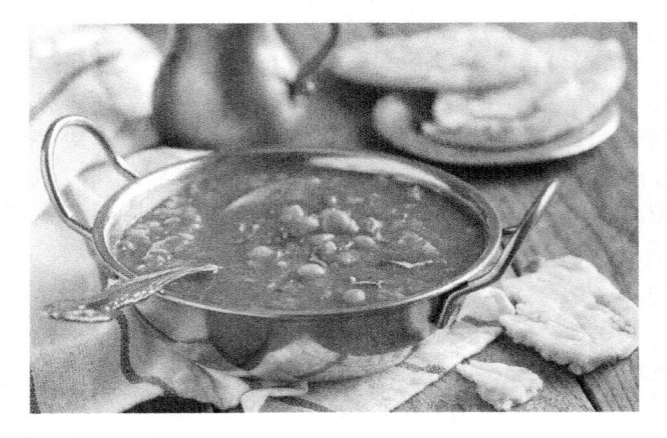

Cooking Time: 1 Hour 20 Minutes
Serving Size: 6–8 Servings

Ingredients

- 3 cups of cooked Garbanzo Beans
- 1 chopped Tomatillo
- 10 chopped Plum Tomatoes
- 1/2 cup of chopped Green Bell Pepper
- 1/2 cup of chopped Red Bell Pepper
- 1/2 cup of minced Onions
- 2 teaspoons of Onion Powder
- 2 teaspoons of Pure Sea Salt
- 1 teaspoon of Sweet Basil
- 1 teaspoon of Cayenne Powder*
- 1 teaspoon of Oregano
- 1/2 teaspoon of Achiote
- 2 teaspoons of Grapeseed Oil
- 1 cup of Spring Water
- Prepared *Sausage Links (see on page 92)*

Cooking Instructions
1. Add Tomatillo, Onions, Bell Peppers, and Grapeseed Oil to a large pot.
2. Sauté vegetables on medium heat for about 4–5 minutes.
3. Put Tomatoes, seasonings*, Garbanzo Beans, and Spring Water in the pot.
4. Stir and bring to a boil.
5. Cook on low heat for about 1 hour. Stir occasionally.
6. Cut the prepared *Sausage Links* into slices. Add them a couple of minutes before the soup is fully cooked.
7. Serve** and enjoy your Spicy Tomato Bean Soup!

Useful Tips

* If you want it to be less spicy, add only 1/2 teaspoon of Cayenne instead.

** You can serve Spicy Tomato Bean Soup with our *Tortillas (see recipe on page 116)* or *Herb Bread (see recipe on page 120)*.

CREAMY CUCUMBER GAZPACHO

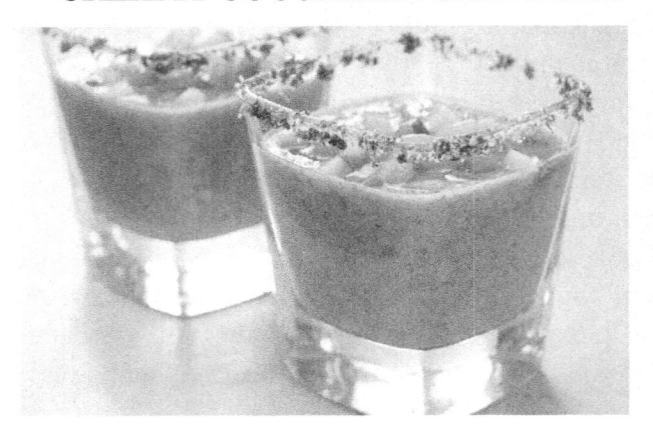

Cooking Time: 15 Minutes
Serving Size: 2 Servings

Ingredients
- 1 Cucumber
- 1 ripe Avocado
- Juice from 1 Key Lime
- 2 handfuls of Basil
- 1–1/4 teaspoons of Pure Sea Salt
- 2 cups of Spring Water

Cooking Instructions
1. Store all ingredients (except Sea Salt) in a refrigerator until cold. Peel the Cucumber and remove all seeds from it.
2. Add all ingredients to a blender and puree them until smooth with some green specks.
3. Pour the mixture into a pot with a lid. Put the soup back in the refrigerator. Allow it to chill about 10 minutes.
4. Serve and garnish with Basil leaves and sliced Cucumber.
5. Serve with *Chickpea "Tofu" (see recipe on page 121)* and enjoy your Creamy Cucumber Gazpacho!

SALADS

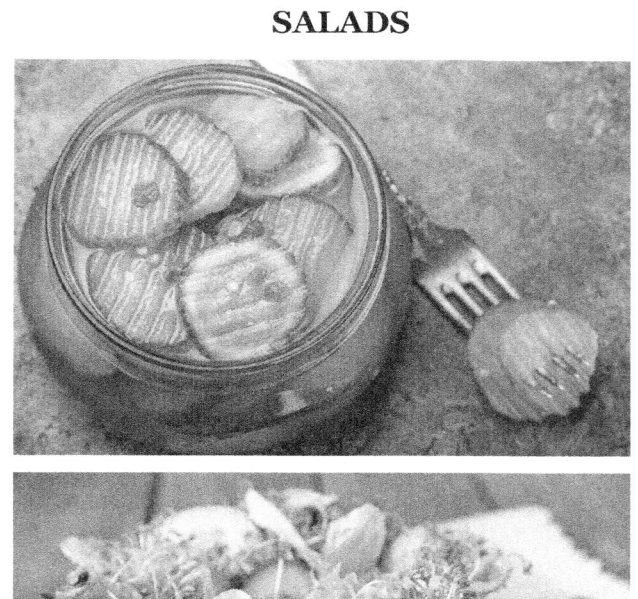

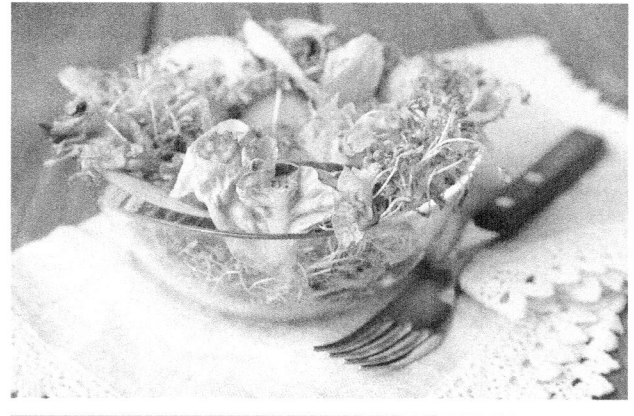

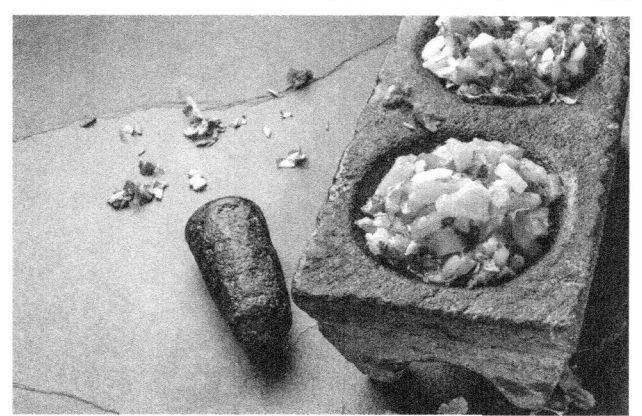

"POTATO" SALAD

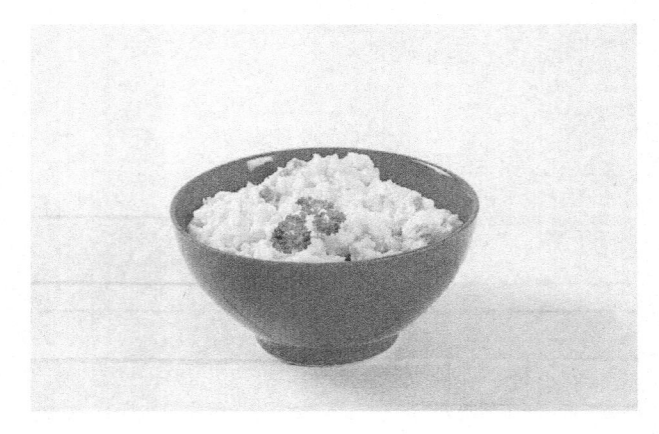

Cooking Time: 20 Minutes + 30 Minutes in the refrigerator
Serving Size: 4 Servings

Ingredients
- 2 cups of cooked Garbanzo Beans
- 1 cup of soaked Brazil Nuts (overnight or at least 4 hours)
- 1/4 cup of diced Green Bell Peppers
- 1/4 cup of diced Onions
- 1 tablespoon of Lime Juice
- 2 teaspoons of Avocado Oil
- 1 teaspoon of Dill
- 1 teaspoon of Onion Powder
- 1 teaspoon of Pure Sea Salt
- 1/2 teaspoon of Sea Moss Gel
- 1/2 teaspoon of Ginger Powder
- 1 cup of Spring Water
- Pinch of Cayenne Powder

Cooking Instructions
1. Put Brazil Nuts, Avocado Oil, Lime Juice, seasonings, and 1/2 cup of Spring Water to a blender.
2. Blend it well for 1 minute.

3. Pour 1/4 cup of Spring Water and Sea Moss Gel to the blender.
4. Mix until smooth consistency. Add extra Spring Water if it is too thick.
5. Put the prepared mixture in a medium-sized bowl.
6. Add Green Bell Peppers and Onions to the bowl and mix well.
7. Let it cool in the refrigerator for 30 minutes before serving.
8. Serve and enjoy your "Potato" Salad!

Useful Tips

* You can serve "Potato" Salad with our *Tortilla Chips (see recipe on page 118) or Tortillas (see recipe on page 116)*.

ZUCCHINI-AND-SQUASH SALAD

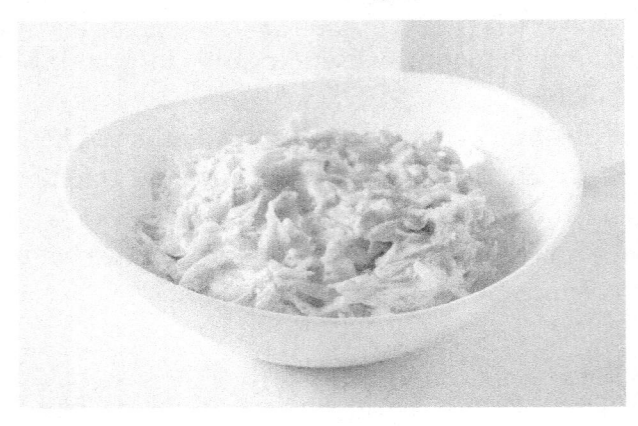

Cooking Time: 30 Minutes + 1 Hour in the refrigerator
Serving Size: 4 Servings

Ingredients
- 2 cups of shredded Zucchini
- 1/2 cup of shredded Butternut Squash
- 1/2 cup of soaked Brazil Nuts (overnight or at least 4 hours)
- 1/4 cup of *Homemade Hempseed Milk (see recipe on page 114)*
- 1/4 cup of chopped Onion
- 1/4 teaspoon of chopped Dates
- 1/2 teaspoon of Sea Moss Gel
- 1/2 teaspoon of Pure Sea Salt
- 1/2 teaspoon of Lime Juice
- 1/2 cup of Spring Water

Cooking Instructions
1. Prepare all ingredients: chop Onions and Dates, shred Butternut Squash and Zucchini.

2. Add Dates, *Homemade Hempseed Milk*, Brazil Nuts, Lime Juice, Sea Moss Gel, Pure Sea Salt and 1/4 cup of Spring Water to a blender. Blend it well for 1 minute.
3. Check the consistency. If it is too thick, add more Spring Water and blend it again.
4. Put vegetables in a medium-sized bowl, add half of the dressing and mix it well. Add more dressing if needed.
5. Allow to cool in a refrigerator for 1 hour before serving.
6. Serve and enjoy your Zucchini-and-Squash Salad!

FRESH SALAD

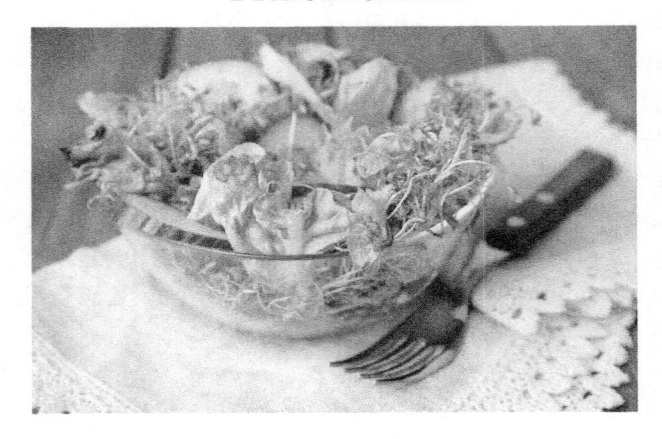

Cooking Time: 5 Minutes
Serving Size: 2 Servings

Ingredients
- 1/2 of sliced Cucumber
- 2 cups of torn Watercress
- 1 tablespoon of Key Lime Juice
- 2 tablespoons of Olive Oil
- Cayenne Powder, to taste
- Pure Sea Salt, to taste

Cooking Instructions
1. Pour Olive Oil and Key Lime Juice into a salad bowl. Mix them well to combine.
2. Slice the Cucumber and add it to the bowl.
3. Tear Watercress and add them to the bowl.
4. Sprinkle Cayenne Powder and Pure Sea Salt on the top according to your liking.
5. Mix it thoroughly.
6. Serve and enjoy your quick Fresh Salad!

QUICK MANGO SALSA

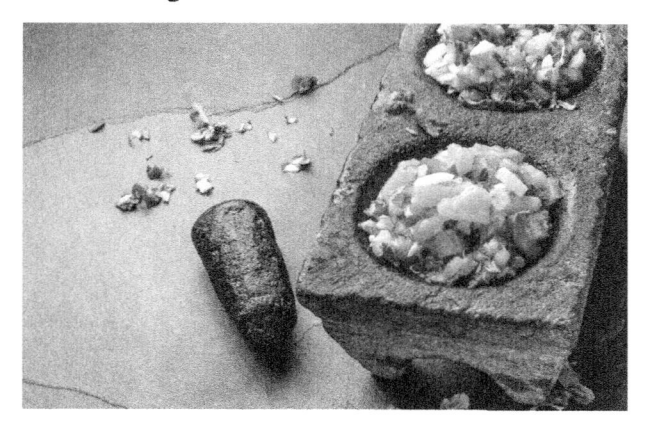

Cooking Time: 15 Minutes
Serving Size: 3 Servings

Ingredients
- 6 Plum Tomatoes
- 1/2 cup of diced Mango
- 1 Tomatillo
- 1/2 cup of diced Red Onions
- 1/4 cup of chopped Green Bell Peppers
- 1/2 cup of Cilantro
- 1 teaspoon of Pure Sea Salt
- 1 teaspoon of Onion Powder
- 1/2 teaspoon of Cayenne Powder
- Juice from half of a Lime

Cooking Instructions
1. Put all ingredients in a food processor (except the Mango).
2. Blend for just 10 seconds.
3. Add Mango to other ingredients, mix it gently using a spoon.
4. Blend 5–10 seconds more, until all ingredients are mixed.
5. Serve with *Tortilla Chips (see on page 118)* and enjoy it!

CHICKPEA SALAD

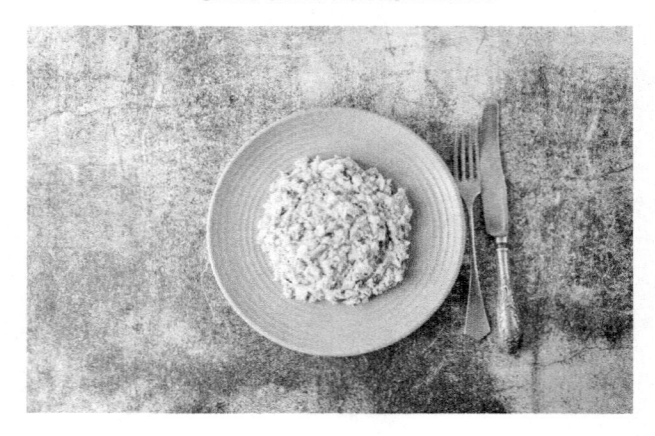

Cooking Time: 20 Minutes + 30–60 minutes in the refrigerator
Serving Size: 2–4 Servings

Ingredients

- 2 cups of cooked Chickpeas
- 2/3 cup of *Hempseed Mayonnaise (see on page 98)*
- 1/4 cup of diced Red Onions
- 1/8 cup of diced Green Bell Peppers
- 1/2 Nori Sheet
- 1 teaspoon of Dill
- 2 teaspoons of Onion Powder
- 1/4 teaspoon of Pure Sea Salt

Cooking Instructions

1. Place Chickpeas into a bowl and mash until desired consistency.
2. Cut Nori Sheet into small pieces and add them to the bowl.
3. Put all remaining ingredients in the bowl and mix it well.
4. Let it cool for 30–60 minutes in a refrigerator before serving.
5. Serve with *Tortilla Chips (see on page 118)* and enjoy it!

PICKLE SALAD

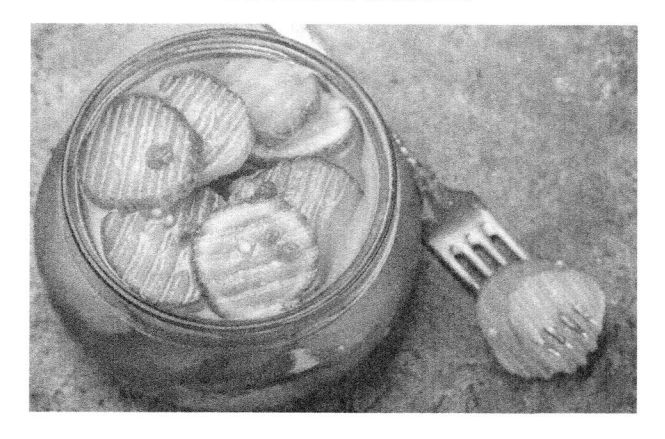

Cooking Time: 20 Minutes + 30 Minutes in the refrigerator
Serving Size: 1 Serving

Ingredients
- 1 cup of sliced Cucumbers
- 1 tablespoon of fresh Dill
- 1 tablespoon of Key Lime Juice
- 1 teaspoon of Coriander
- 1 teaspoon of Pure Sea Salt
- 1/2 teaspoon of Crushed Red Pepper
- 1/2 cup of Spring Water

Cooking Instructions
1. Cut off the ends of Cucumbers and slice them using a crinkle tool.
2. Crush the coriander using a pestle.
3. Put slices of Cucumbers, Coriander, and all other ingredients in a jar with a lid. Shake it well.
4. Let it infuse for 6–8 hours; shake it every 1–2 hours.
5. Serve and enjoy your Pickle Salad!

SAUTÉED KALE

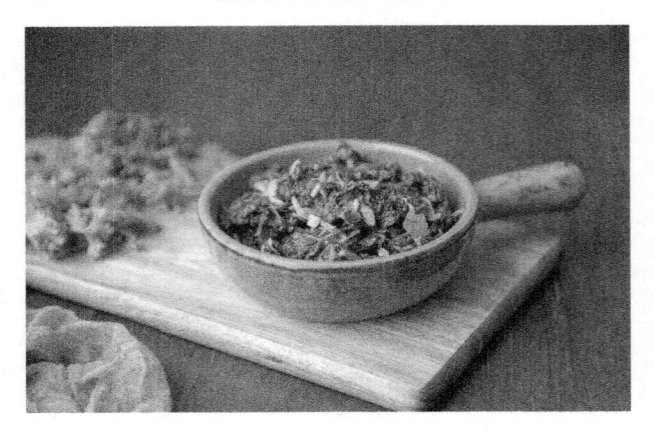

Cooking Time: 15 Minutes
Serving Size: 4 Servings

Ingredients
- 1 bunch of Kale
- 1/4 cup of minced Onions
- 1/4 cup of minced Red Pepper
- 1/4 teaspoon of Pure Sea Salt
- 1 teaspoon of Crushed Red Pepper flakes
- 2 tablespoons of Grapeseed Oil
- 1/4 teaspoon of Pure Sea Salt

Cooking Instructions
1. Fold rinsed Kale leaves in half and cut off the stems.
2. Dice Kale into small pieces. Spin in a salad spinner* until dry. If you don't have it, just wait until the Kale is dry.
3. Take a wok, add Grapeseed Oil, and warm it on high heat.
4. Add minced Onions and Red Pepper to the wok and sauté on medium heat for 2–3 minutes.
5. Add Kale leaves and Pure Sea Salt to the pan. Cover it with a lid. Reduce to low heat and cook for about 5 minutes.
6. Spread crushed Pepper flakes and mix thoroughly. Cover with a lid and cook for 3 minutes. Serve and enjoy it!

MAIN DISHES

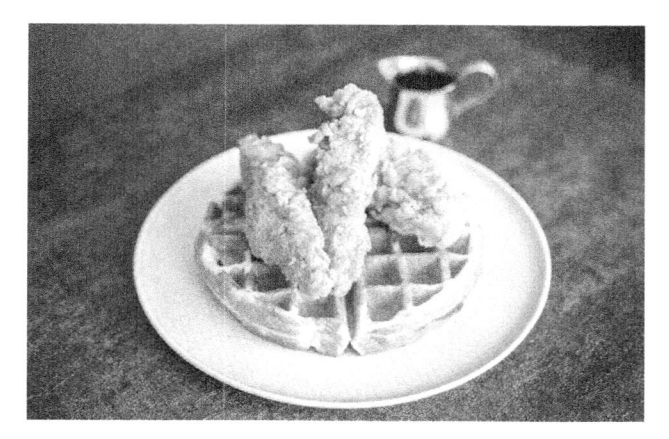

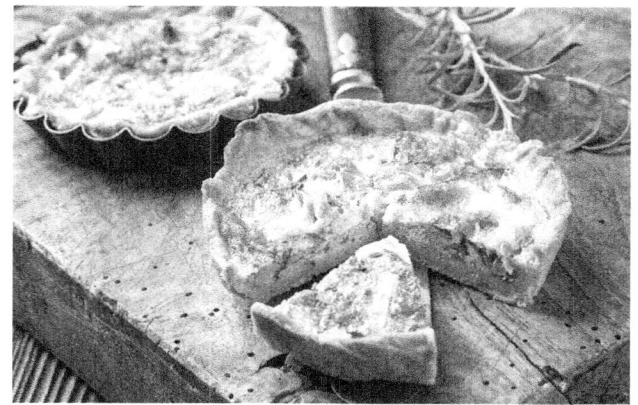

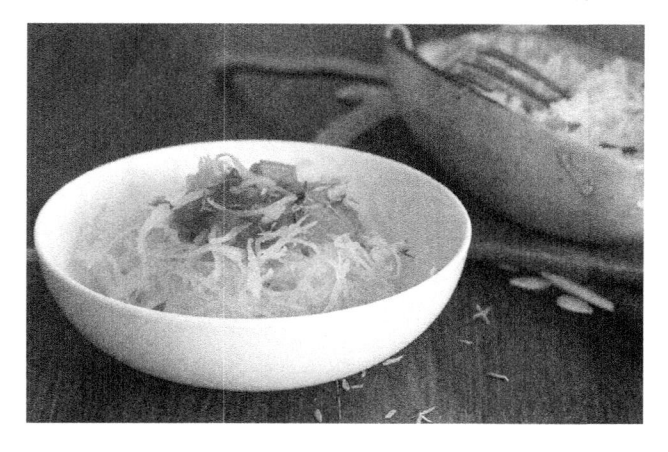

VEGETARIAN PIZZA

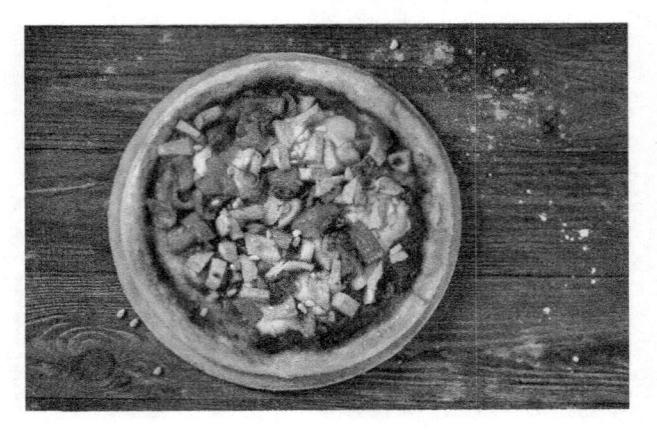

Cooking Time: 45 Minutes
Serving Size: 4–6 Servings

Ingredients

Crust
- 1–1/2 cups of Spelt Flour*
- 2 teaspoons of Sesame Seeds
- 2 teaspoons of Grapeseed Oil
- 2 teaspoons of Agave Syrup
- 1 teaspoon of Pure Sea Salt
- 1 teaspoon of Oregano
- 1 teaspoon of Onion Powder
- 1 cup of Spring Water

Filling
- *Tomato Pizza Sauce (see recipe on page 99)*
- *"Cheese" Sauce (see recipe on page 100)*
- Diced Mushrooms
- Diced Bell Peppers
- Chopped Onions

Cooking Instructions
1. Preheat your oven to 400°F.
2. Mix all crust ingredients with just 1/2 cup of Spring Water in a medium-sized bowl. Add Spring Water slowly, kneading the dough until you can form a ball.
3. Take a baking sheet and coat it with some Grapeseed Oil.
4. Roll out the dough and put it on the baking sheet.
5. Brush the dough top with Grapeseed Oil and make holes using a fork.
6. Bake the crust for about 12–15 minutes.
7. Add *Tomato Pizza Sauce*, Mushrooms, Onions, Peppers, and *"Cheese" Sauce* on the baked crust.
8. Continue baking for more 15–20 minutes.
9. Serve and enjoy your Vegetarian Pizza!

Useful Tips
* If you don't have Spelt Flour, you can add Kamut Flour instead.

MUSHROOM GRAVY

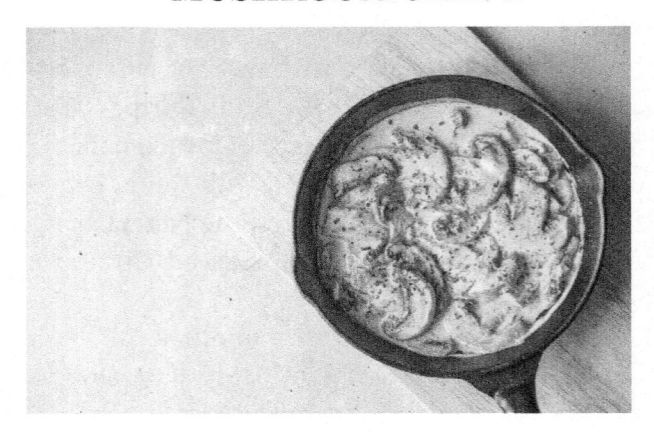

Cooking Time: 40 Minutes
Serving Size: 3–4 Servings

Ingredients
- 1/2 cup of sliced Mushrooms
- 1/2 cup of chopped Onions
- 3 tablespoons of Chickpea Flour
- 1 teaspoon of Onion Powder
- 1 teaspoon of Pure Sea Salt
- 1/2 teaspoon of Thyme
- 1/2 teaspoon of Oregano
- 1/4 teaspoon of Cayenne Powder
- 2 tablespoons of Grapeseed Oil
- 2–3 cups of Spring Water

Cooking Instructions
1. Put a frying pan on high heat and lightly grease it with Grapeseed Oil.
2. Reduce to medium heat. Add chopped Onions, sliced Mushrooms, and sauté for 1–2 minutes.
3. Add all seasonings and spices (except Cayenne Powder). Sauté for 5–6 minutes.

4. Pour 2 cups of Spring Water in and add Cayenne Powder.
5. Mix everything well and bring to a boil.
6. Add Chickpea Flour, stirring it slowly and whisking to avoid making lumps.
7. Continue to cook to a boil, adding remaining Spring Water if needed.
8. Serve and enjoy your Mushroom Gravy!

EGG FOO YUNG

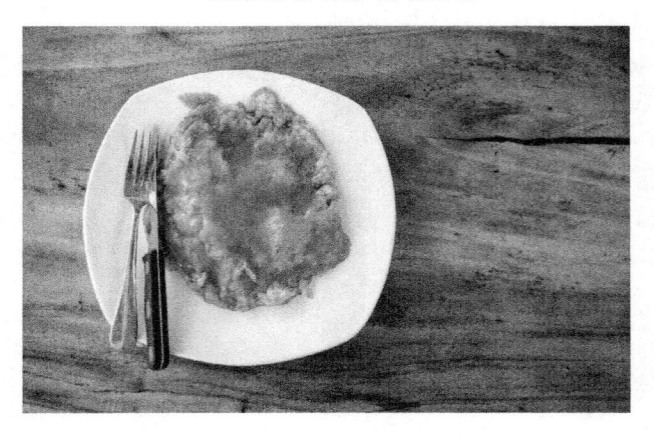

Cooking Time: 40 Minutes
Serving Size: 3–4 Servings

Ingredients

- 3 cups of cooked *Spaghetti Squash (see recipe on page 72)*
- 1 cup of diced Butternut Squash
- 2 cups of sliced Mushrooms
- 1/2 cup of chopped White and Red Onions
- 1/2 cup of chopped Green Onions
- 1/2 cup of diced Green & Red Bell Peppers
- 3/4 cup of Chickpea Flour
- 1 teaspoon of Onion Powder
- 1 teaspoon of Oregano
- 1 teaspoon of Basil
- 1 teaspoon of Pure Sea Salt
- 1/2 teaspoon of Cayenne Powder
- 1/8 teaspoon of Ginger Powder
- 2 teaspoons of Grapeseed Oil
- 1 cup of Spring Water

Cooking Instructions
1. Add Spring Water, Chickpea Flour, and seasonings in a large bowl. Mix together.
2. Add chopped vegetables to the bowl and mix. Then add prepared Spaghetti Squash and mix with hands until well mixed.
3. Place a large skillet on high heat, lightly grease it with Grapeseed Oil, and put in 1/2 cup of the mixture.
4. Form patties and cook for about 3–4 minutes on each side until golden-brown.
5. Serve* and enjoy your Egg Foo Yung!

Useful Tips

* You can serve it with our *Orange-Ginger Sauce (see recipe on page 95)* or *Mushroom Gravy (see recipe on page 62)*.

TEFF PATTIES

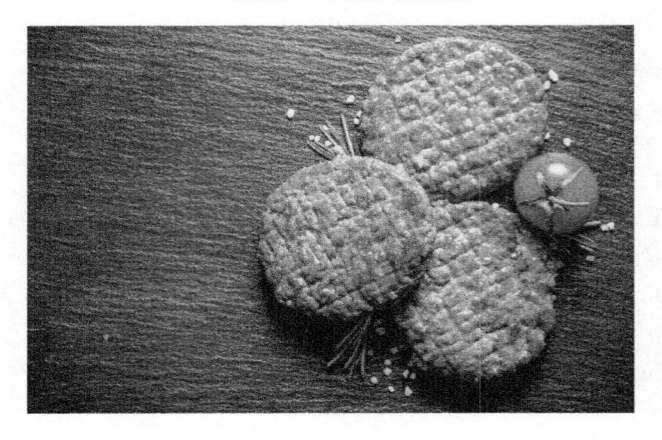

Cooking Time: 40 Minutes
Serving Size: 3–4 Servings

Ingredients

- 1-1/2 cups of cooked Teff Grain
- 1/2 cup of Garbanzo Bean Flour
- 1/4 cup of chopped Onions
- 1 tablespoon of Onion Powder
- 1 tablespoon of diced Green Bell Peppers
- 1 tablespoon of diced Red Bell Peppers
- 2 teaspoons of Ground Sage
- 1 teaspoon of Basil
- 1 teaspoon of Oregano
- 1 teaspoon of Fennel Powder
- 1 teaspoon of Pure Sea Salt
- 1/2 teaspoon of Crushed Red Pepper
- 1/2 teaspoon of Dill
- 2–3 tablespoons of Grapeseed Oil

Cooking Instructions

1. Put your skillet pan on medium-high heat, add 1 tablespoon Grapeseed Oil.

2. Add diced Bell Peppers and chopped Onions into the warm pan and sauté them for 2–3 minutes.
3. Put sautéed vegetables, Teff Grain, seasonings, and spices in a large bowl. Mix them well. Continue mixing, and add Garbanzo Bean Flour last.
4. Put a skillet on medium heat, coat with 1–2 tablespoons of Grapeseed Oil.
5. Form patties from the prepared mixture and cook for 3–4 minutes on each side until brown.
6. Serve* and enjoy your Teff Patties!

Useful Tips

* You can serve it with our *"Cheese" Sauce (see recipe on page 100), Spicy Tomato Sauce (see recipe on page 96), Orange-Ginger Sauce (see recipe on page 95), Hempseed Mayonnaise (see recipe on page 98),* or *Mushroom Gravy (see recipe on page 62).*

WAFFLES & VEGGIE "CHICKEN"

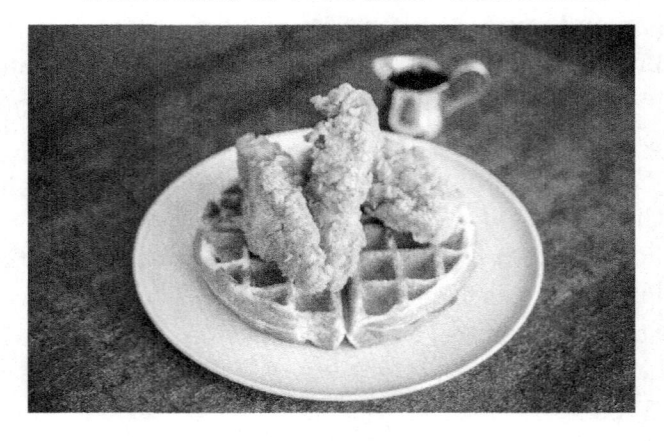

Cooking Time: 40 Minutes
Serving Size: 2 Servings

Ingredients
<u>Waffles</u>
- 2 cups of Spelt Flour*
- 1 cup of *Homemade Hempseed Milk (see recipe on page 114)*
- 1/4 cup of Agave Syrup
- 2 teaspoons of Sea Moss Gel (optional)
- 3 tablespoons of Grapeseed Oil
- 1/4 teaspoon of Pure Sea Salt
- 1 cup of Spring Water

<u>Veggie "Chicken"</u>
- 1–2 bunches of Oyster Mushrooms
- 3/4 cup of prepared *Waffle Batter*
- 3/4 cup of Chickpea Flour
- 2 teaspoons of Onion Powder
- 1 teaspoon of Oregano
- 1 teaspoon of Basil
- 1/2 teaspoon of Cayenne Powder

- 1/2 teaspoon of Pure Sea Salt

Cooking Instructions
1. Put all ingredients with just 1/2 cup of Spring Water in a large bowl. Mix it well. If the batter is too thick, add more Spring Water.
2. Set aside a 3/4 cup of prepared waffle batter.
3. Take a waffle maker, brush it with some Grapeseed Oil and cook every waffle for 3–5 minutes.
4. Prepare the Oyster Mushrooms, remove them from the base, wash, and clean.
5. Put Chickpea Flour and half of the seasonings (intended for Veggie "Chicken") in a container with a lid. Mix them well.
6. Add the Oyster Mushrooms to the container, cover with a lid, and gently toss them.
7. Add the other part of the seasonings to the remaining waffle batter (3/4 cup), some Spring Water, and mix. Coat Oyster Mushrooms with this mixture.
8. Put your skillet on high heat, add 3 tablespoons of Grapeseed Oil, reduce to medium-high heat, and cook coated Mushrooms for 3–4 minutes, flipping sometimes.
9. Serve*** and enjoy your Waffles with Veggie "Chicken"!

Useful Tips
* If you don't have Spelt Flour, you can add Kamut Flour instead.
** If you don't have prepared *Homemade Hempseed Milk*, you can add *Homemade Walnut Milk (see recipe on page 107)* instead.
*** You can serve it with our *"Cheese" Sauce (see recipe on page 100)*, *Spicy Tomato Sauce (see recipe on page 96)*, *"Garlic" Sauce (see recipe on page 102)*, *Hempseed Mayonnaise (see recipe on page 98)*, or *Orange-Ginger Sauce (see recipe on page 95)*.

MUSHROOM STRIPS

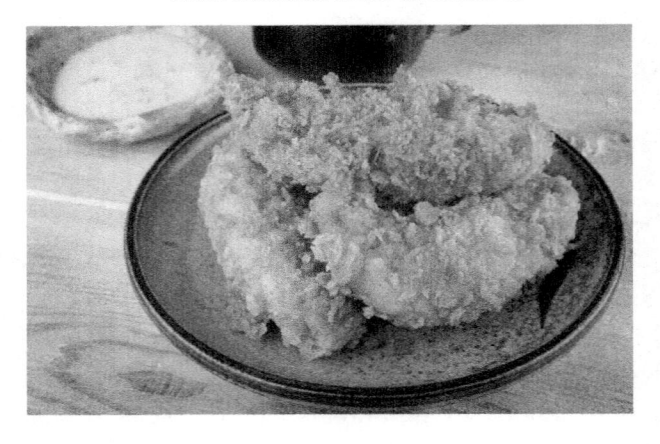

Cooking Time: 50 Minutes + 1 Hour for marinating
Serving Size: 3–4 Servings

Ingredients
- 2–6 Portabella Mushrooms*
- 1–1/2 cups of Spelt Flour**
- 1–1/2 cups of *Aquafaba (see recipe on page 108)*
- 2 teaspoons of Basil
- 2 teaspoons of Sage
- 2 teaspoons of Oregano
- 2 teaspoons of Ginger Powder
- 2 teaspoons of Onion Powder
- 2 teaspoons of Pure Sea Salt
- 1 teaspoon of Allspice
- 1 teaspoon of Cayenne Powder
- 2–3 tablespoons of Grapeseed Oil

Cooking Instructions
1. Cut Portabella Mushroom* caps into 1/2-inch slices and put them in a large container. You can cut off the stems to make slices look like nuggets.

2. Put *Aquafaba*, 1 teaspoon of Grapeseed Oil, and half of the seasonings in the container and mix all together. Let it marinate for 1 hour.
3. Mix together the rest of the seasonings, Spelt Flour** and Mushroom mixture.
4. Preheat your oven to 400°F.
5. Take a baking pan, cover with a piece of parchment paper, and grease it with some Grapeseed Oil. Put Mushroom pieces on it.
6. Bake for about 15 minutes, flip them, and continue cooking for an additional 15 minutes.
7. Serve*** and enjoy your Mushroom Strips!

Useful Tips

* If you don't have/like Portabella Mushrooms, you can use White or Oyster Mushrooms instead. Adjust *Aquafaba* and flour according to the amount of Mushrooms.

** If you don't have Spelt Flour, you can add Kamut Flour instead.

*** You can serve it with our *"Cheese" Sauce (see recipe on page 100), Tomato Pizza Sauce (see recipe on page 99), Orange-Ginger Sauce (see recipe on page 95),* or *Hempseed Mayonnaise (see recipe on page 98).*

SPAGHETTI SQUASH

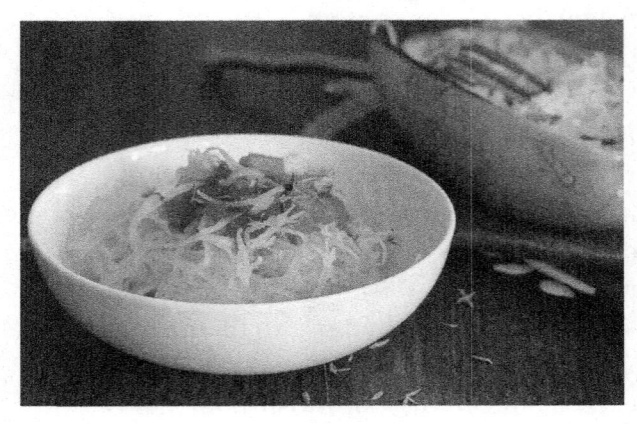

Cooking Time: 40 Minutes
Serving Size: 4 Servings

Ingredients
- 1 Spaghetti Squash
- 2 teaspoons of Grapeseed Oil
- 1/2 teaspoon of Pure Sea Salt
- 1/2 teaspoon of Onion Powder
- 1/4 teaspoon of Cayenne Powder

Cooking Instructions
1. Preheat your oven to 375°F.
2. Cut off the ends of Spaghetti Squash and divide it in half.
3. Take out the seeds and insides from the Squash.
4. Add Grapeseed Oil and seasoning to the Squash halves. Lightly coat them inside and outside.
5. Bake the halves for about 30–35 minutes. The outside part of the Squash should become tender; if not, bake them longer.
6. Let it cool for a couple of minutes. Take a fork and scrape the insides out into a bowl.
7. Serve and enjoy Spaghetti Squash!

WALNUT FILLING

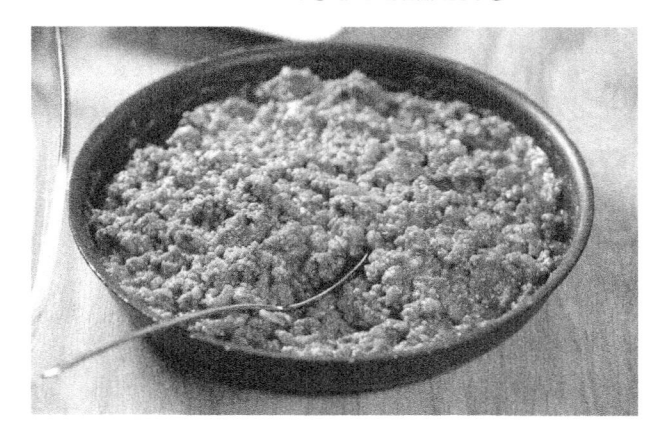

Cooking Time: 10 Minutes + 6–8 Hours for soaking
Serving Size: 1–2 Servings

Ingredients
- 1 cup of Walnuts
- 1 Plum Tomato
- 1/2 teaspoon of Onion Powder
- 1/2 teaspoon of Cayenne Powder
- 1/2 teaspoon of Ginger
- 1/2 teaspoon of Pure Sea Salt
- 1 teaspoon of Grapeseed Oil
- Spring Water

Cooking Instructions
1. Put Walnuts in a small bowl, cover with Spring Water, and soak for about 6–8 hours. Refrigerate if needed.
2. Add soaked Walnuts, Plum Tomato, spices, and seasonings in a food processor.
3. Pulse until ingredients are mixed.
4. Serve* it raw or sauté with other favorite vegetables.
5. Enjoy your Walnut Filling! You can serve it with burritos, wraps, tacos, nachos, and more!

ZUCCHINI BACON

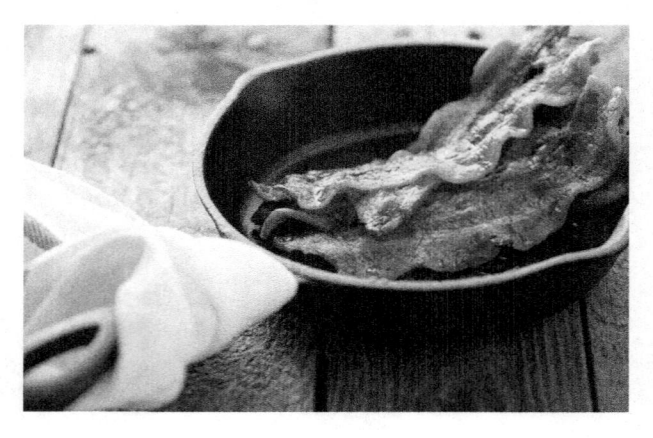

Cooking Time: 30 Minutes + 1 Hour for marinating
Serving Size: 2–3 Servings

Ingredients

- 3 medium Zucchinis
- 1/4 cup of Date Sugar
- 2 tablespoons of Agave Syrup
- 1 tablespoon of Onion Powder
- 1 tablespoon of Pure Sea Salt
- 1 teaspoon of Liquid Smoke
- 1/2 teaspoon of Ginger Powder
- 1/2 teaspoon of Cayenne Powder
- 1/4 cup of Spring Water
- 1 teaspoon of Grapeseed Oil

Cooking Instructions

1. Put all ingredients (except Grapeseed Oil and Zucchinis) in a saucepan and cook on low heat until dissolved.
2. Cut off the ends of Zucchinis and make strips using a potato peeler.
3. Pour saucepan mixture in a large bowl and add Zucchini strips. Allow to marinate for 40–60 minutes.

4. Preheat your oven to 400°F.
5. Take a baking pan, cover with a piece of parchment paper, and grease it with some Grapeseed Oil.
6. Place Zucchini strips on the baking pan and cook for 10 minutes.
7. Flip them over and continue cooking for 3–4 more minutes.
8. Serve* and enjoy your Zucchini Bacon!

Useful Tips

* You can serve it with our *"Cheese" Sauce (see recipe on page 100), Tomato Pizza Sauce (see recipe on page 99), Orange-Ginger Sauce (see recipe on page 95),* or *Hempseed Mayonnaise (see recipe on page 98).*

HOMEMADE PASTA

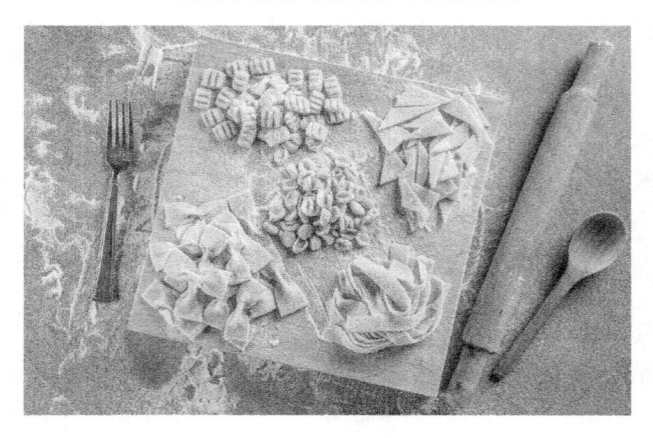

Cooking Time: 50 Minutes
Serving Size: 4 Servings

Ingredients
- 2 cups of Spelt Flour*
- 2 tablespoons of Grapeseed Oil
- 3/4 cup of warm Spring Water
- 1/2 teaspoon of Pure Sea Salt

Cooking Instructions
1. In a large bowl, mix together warm Spring Water, 1 cup of Spelt Flour*, and Pure Sea Salt until it can be shaped into a ball.
2. Spread extra flour on your workspace.
3. Knead the dough for 6–8 minutes.
4. Make a ball and cover it first with flour then with plastic wrap. Set aside for 15–20 minutes.
5. Unwrap the dough and divide it into 4 equal parts.
6. Take 1 part you are going to work with. Re-wrap the 3 other parts.
7. Roll the dough out in one direction a couple of times with a rolling pin, then flip it and repeat the rolling process. Remember to add more flour while flipping.

8. Cut the dough into individual pieces of pasta using a pastry cutter. Look at the picture and you will see some examples.
9. Repeat steps 6, 7, and 8 with the remaining dough.
10. Pour Spring Water and Pure Sea Salt into a large pot and bring to a boil.
11. Cook pasta in the boiling water for 1–2 minutes then strain.
12. Serve** and enjoy your Homemade Pasta!

Useful Tips
* If you don't have Spelt Flour, you can add Kamut Flour instead.
** You can serve it with our *"Cheese" Sauce (see recipe on page 100)* or *Spicy Tomato Sauce (see recipe on page 96)*.

QUICHE

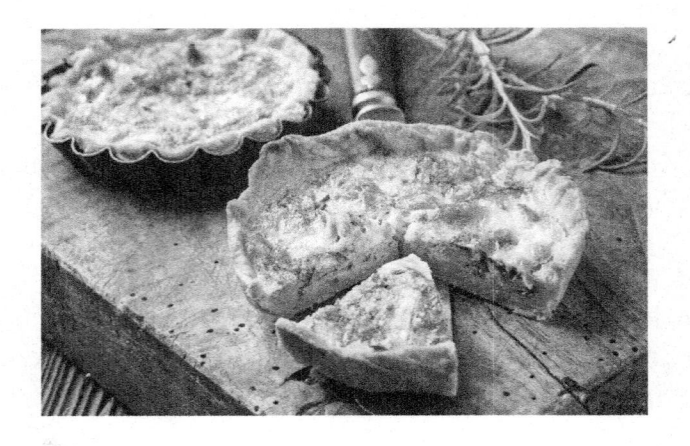

Cooking Time: 1 Hour 30 Minutes
Serving Size: 6–8 Servings

Ingredients
Crust
- 1 cup of Spelt Flour*
- 1 teaspoon of Oregano
- 1 teaspoon of Onion Powder
- 1 teaspoon of Basil
- 1 teaspoon of Pure Sea Salt
- 1 cup of Spring Water

Filling
- 2 cups of sliced Mushrooms
- 1 cup of Garbanzo Bean Flour
- 1 cup of *"Cheese" Sauce (see recipe on page 100)*
- 1 cup of chopped Kale
- 3/4 cup of *Aquafaba (see recipe on page 108)*
- 3/4 cup of *Hempseed Milk (see recipe on page 114)***
- 1/2 cup of diced Yellow, Green, and Red Bell Peppers
- 1/2 cup of chopped White and Red Onions
- 1 tablespoon of Sea Moss Gel

- 1 tablespoon of *"Garlic" Sauce (see recipe on page 102)*
- 1 tablespoon of Onion Powder
- 1 teaspoon of Basil
- 1 teaspoon of Oregano
- 1 teaspoon of Pure Sea Salt
- 1/4 teaspoon of Cayenne Powder

Cooking Instructions
1. Mix together seasonings and Spelt Flour* (for the crust). Pour in Spring Water and knead the dough until the ball can be formed.
2. Prepare your workplace, spread some flour, and roll out the dough. It should fit into a pie pan. Add more flour after every time you flip the dough.
3. Lightly grease the pie pan with some Grapeseed Oil, fit rolled dough into the pan, and cut off the edges.
4. Make the quiche filling. Add *Aquafaba, Homemade Hempseed Milk**,* Garbanzo Bean Flour, *Garlic Sauce*, seasonings, and Sea Moss Gel to a blender and mix it well until smooth.
5. Preheat your oven to 350°F.
6. Mix together chopped Bell Peppers, Onions, Kale, and Mushrooms in a large bowl.
7. Put mixed vegetables on the dough, then pour *Cheese Sauce* and prepared quiche filling.
8. Place foil on the top of the pie and bake for about 50 minutes. Remove the foil and continue cooking for more 10 minutes.
9. Serve and enjoy your Quiche!

Useful Tips
* If you don't have Spelt Flour, you can add Garbanzo Bean Flour instead.
** If you don't have prepared *Hempseed Milk*, you can add *Homemade Walnut Milk (see recipe on page 107)* instead.

VEGGIE ALFREDO

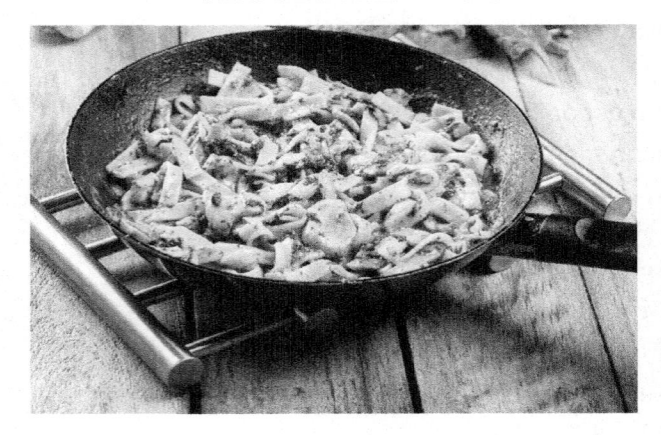

Cooking Time: 20 Minutes
Serving Size: 4–6 Servings

Ingredients

- 5 cups of *Homemade Pasta (see recipe on page 76)*
- 1 cup of *"Cheese" Sauce (see recipe on page 100)*
- 8–10 chopped Mushrooms
- 1 chopped Red Bell Pepper
- 1 chopped Orange Bell Pepper
- 1 chopped Zucchini Squash
- 1 chopped Summer Squash
- 1 chopped Onion
- 1/2 teaspoon of Basil
- 1/2 teaspoon of Oregano
- 1/2 teaspoon of Onion Powder
- 1/4 teaspoon of Cayenne Powder
- 1 teaspoon of Pure Sea Salt
- 1 tablespoon of Grapeseed Oil

Cooking Instructions
1. Bring water to a boil in a medium pot, cook *Homemade Pasta* for 1–2 minutes, and drain it.
2. Chop up all vegetables. Put a skillet on medium-high heat, add some Grapeseed Oil, chopped vegetables, seasonings, and herbs.
3. Sauté the mixture for 2–3 minutes on medium heat.
4. Add cooked pasta and *Cheese Sauce* into the skillet.
5. Mix all of them and sauté for 1 minute.
6. Serve and enjoy your Veggie Alfredo!

BUTTERNUT SQUASH FRIES

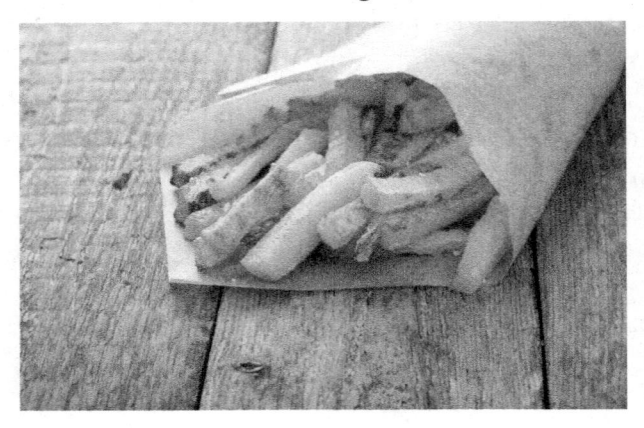

Cooking Time: 25 Minutes
Serving Size: 4–6 Servings

Ingredients
- 1/2 of Butternut Squash
- 1/2 cup of chopped Onion
- 3 tablespoons of Grapeseed Oil
- 1 teaspoon of Pure Sea Salt
- 1 teaspoon of Onion Powder
- 1/2 teaspoon of Cayenne Powder

Cooking Instructions
1. Cut off the ends of Butternut Squash. Remove the skin using a peeler.
2. Cut the vegetable in half at the neck, then cut the body in half.
3. Remove the seeds by using a spoon.
4. Cut the body of Butternut Squash into 1/2-inch sticks. Chop Onion into small pieces.
5. Put a skillet on high heat and add Grapeseed Oil.
6. Add chopped Onion and Butternut Squash sticks into a hot skillet and cook for 8–10 minutes on medium heat or until golden-brown.

7. Spread Pure Sea Salt, Cayenne Powder, Onion Powder, or other seasonings according to your liking.
8. Serve* and enjoy your Butternut Squash Fries!

Useful Tips

* You can serve it with our *"Cheese" Sauce (see recipe on page 100), Tomato Pizza Sauce (see recipe on page 99), Orange-Ginger Sauce (see recipe on page 95),* or *Hempseed Mayonnaise (see recipe on page 98).*

VEGETABLE QUINOA

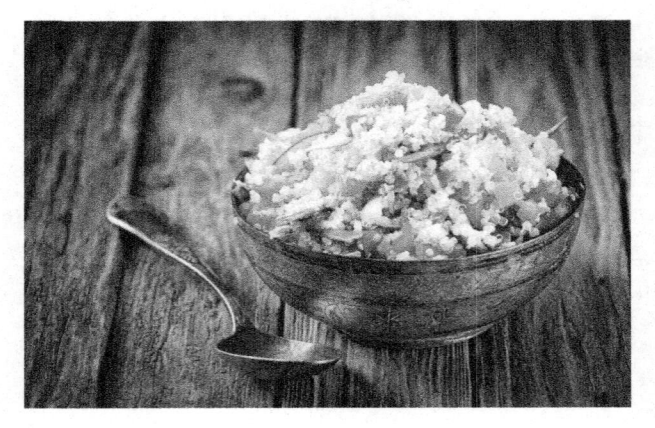

Cooking Time: 20 Minutes
Serving Size: 6–8 Servings

Ingredients

- 4 cups of cooked Quinoa
- 1 cup of chopped Zucchini
- 1/4 cup of diced Yellow Bell Peppers
- 1/4 cup of diced Green Bell Peppers
- 1/4 cup of diced Red Bell Peppers
- 1 diced Plum Tomato
- 1/2 cup of diced Red Onion
- 2 tablespoons of Grapeseed Oil
- 1 tablespoon of Onion Powder
- 2 teaspoons of Pure Sea Salt
- 1 teaspoon of Oregano
- 1 teaspoon of Basil
- 1/2 teaspoon of Cayenne Powder
- 1/2 cup of Spring Water

Cooking Instructions
1. Put a large skillet on high heat and add Grapeseed Oil.
2. Place all diced/chopped vegetables and seasonings into the skillet and sauté for 8–10 minutes.
3. Pour Spring Water in and add Quinoa. Cook for more 5 minutes.
4. Serve and enjoy your Vegetable Quinoa!

ZUCCHINI PATTIES

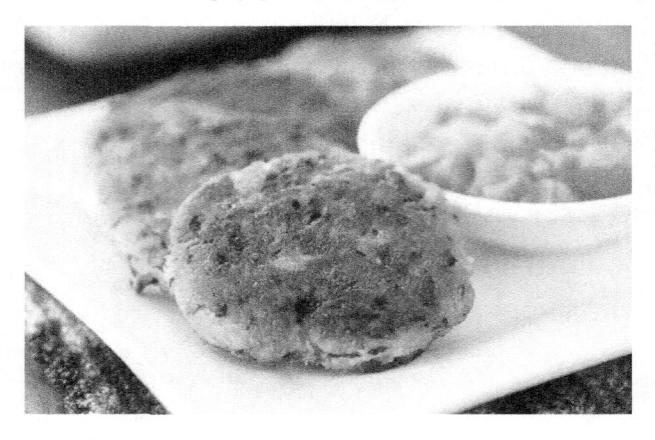

Cooking Time: 50 Minutes
Serving Size: 2 Servings

Ingredients

- 2–3 Zucchinis
- 1/2 cup of Chickpea Flour
- 1/4 cup of *Homemade Hempseed Milk (see recipe on page 114)**
- 1/4 cup of diced Green Onions
- 1/4 cup of diced Onions
- 1 teaspoon of Pure Sea Salt
- 1 teaspoon of Onion Powder
- 1 teaspoon of Parsley
- 1 teaspoon of Oregano
- 1/2 teaspoon of Cayenne Powder
- 2 tablespoons of Grapeseed Oil

Cooking Instructions

1. Shred the Zucchini with a grater.
2. Squeeze the moisture out with a strainer.
3. Add Zucchini, *Hempseed Milk**, Onions, Chickpea Flour, and seasonings in a bowl and mix them together.

4. Put a skillet on medium heat and add some Grapeseed Oil.
5. Put 1/3 cup of the zucchini mixture on the warm skillet and pat it down using a spatula.
6. Cook for 3–5 minutes on each side.
7. Serve** and enjoy your Zucchini Patties!

Useful Tips

* If you don't have *Homemade Hempseed Milk*, add *Homemade Walnut Milk (see recipe on page 107)* instead.

** You can serve it with our *"Cheese" Sauce (see recipe on page 100), Tomato Pizza Sauce (see recipe on page 99), Orange-Ginger Sauce (see recipe on page 95),* or *Hempseed Mayonnaise (see recipe on page 98).*

MASHED BURROS

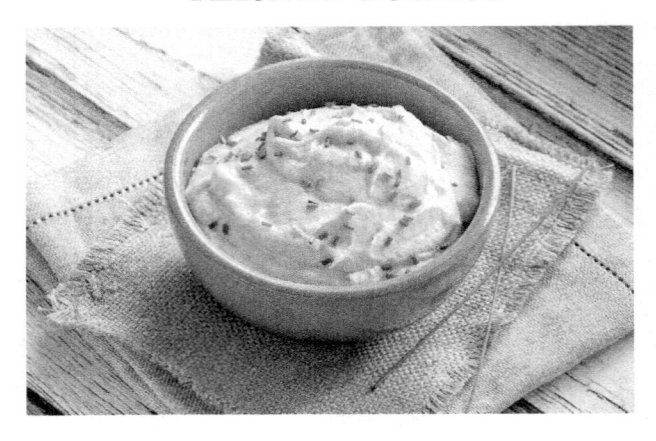

Cooking Time: 40 Minutes
Serving Size: 4–6 Servings

Ingredients
- 6–8 green Burro Bananas*
- 1 cup of *Homemade Hempseed Milk (see recipe on page 114)***
- 1/4 cup of diced Green Onions
- 2 teaspoons of Pure Sea Salt
- 2 teaspoons of Onion Powder
- Spring Water, if needed

Cooking Instructions
1. Cut off the ends of Burro Bananas*, remove the skin, and add bananas to a food processor.
2. Put seasonings and *Homemade Hempseed Milk*** in the food processor. Blend it well for about 2 minutes. Add some Spring Water if the mixture is too thick.
3. Add banana mixture and diced Onions to a saucepan.
4. Cook for about 30 minutes on low heat, stirring occasionally. Pour extra Spring Water if it becomes too thick.
5. Serve*** and enjoy your Mashed Burros!

Useful Tips

* If you don't have green Burro Bananas, add 2 cups of cooked Garbanzo Beans instead.

** If you don't have *Homemade Hempseed Milk*, add *Homemade Walnut Milk (see recipe on page 107)* instead.

*** You can serve it with our *Mushroom Gravy (see recipe on page 62)*.

BAKED BEANS

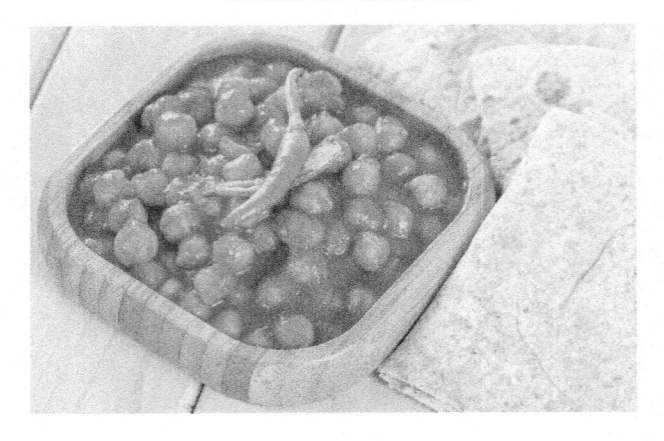

Cooking Time: 1 Hour 40 Minutes
Serving Size: 4–6 Servings

Ingredients
- 5–6 Plum Tomatoes
- 3 cups of cooked Garbanzo Beans
- 1/4 cup of diced Green Bell Peppers
- 1/4 cup of diced Onions
- 1/2 cup of Date Syrup*
- 3 tablespoons of Agave
- 2 teaspoons of Onion Powder
- 2 teaspoons of Pure Sea Salt
- 1/2 teaspoon of Ground Ginger
- 1/4 teaspoon of Cayenne Powder
- 1/8 teaspoon of Cloves

Cooking Instructions
1. Add Plum Tomatoes, Date Syrup, Agave, and seasonings to a blender and blend them until it's a smooth consistency.
2. Put tomato mixture, Bell Peppers, Onions, and cooked Garbanzo Beans to a saucepan.

3. Cook on medium heat for about 20 minutes, stirring occasionally.
4. Reduce to low heat and simmer for about 1 hour.
5. Serve and enjoy your Baked Beans!

Useful Tips
* If you don't have Date Syrup, add 1/4 cup of Date Sugar instead. Cook them with Beans.

SAUSAGE LINKS

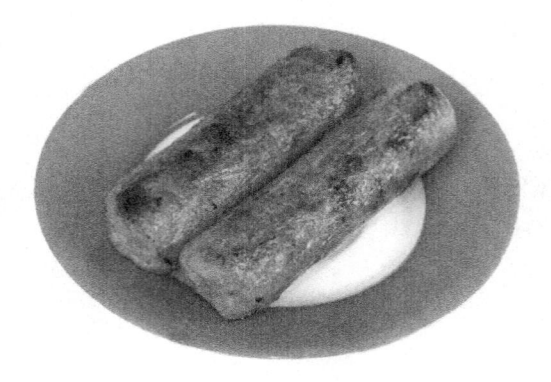

Cooking Time: 30 Minutes
Serving Size: 8–10 Servings

Ingredients
- 1 quartered Plum Tomato
- 1 cup of quartered Mushrooms
- 1/2 cup of Garbanzo Bean Flour
- 2 cups of cooked Garbanzo Beans
- 1/2 cup of chopped Onion
- 1 teaspoon of Basil
- 1 teaspoon of Dill
- 1 tablespoon of Onion Powder
- 1 teaspoon of Ground Sage
- 1 teaspoon of Oregano
- 1 teaspoon of Pure Sea Salt
- 1/2 teaspoon Ground Cloves
- 1/2 teaspoon of Cayenne Powder
- 2 tablespoons of Grapeseed Oil

Cooking Instructions
1. Put all the ingredients (except the Grapeseed Oil and Garbanzo Bean Flour) into your food processor.

2. Blend it for 15 seconds.
3. Add the Garbanzo Bean Flour to the prepared mixture and blend for 30 more seconds until well combined.
4. Put the mixture into a piping bag and cut a small piece from the bottom corner.
5. Add Grapeseed Oil to a skillet and warm on high heat.
6. Reduce to medium heat. Squeeze out the prepared mixture into the pan to form sausages.
7. Cook them for about 3–4 minutes on all sides. Turn carefully to prevent them from falling apart.
8. Serve* and enjoy your Sausage Links!

Useful Tips

* You can serve it with our *"Cheese" Sauce (see recipe on page 100), Tomato Pizza Sauce (see recipe on page 99)* or *Hempseed Mayonnaise (see recipe on page 98).*

SAUCES

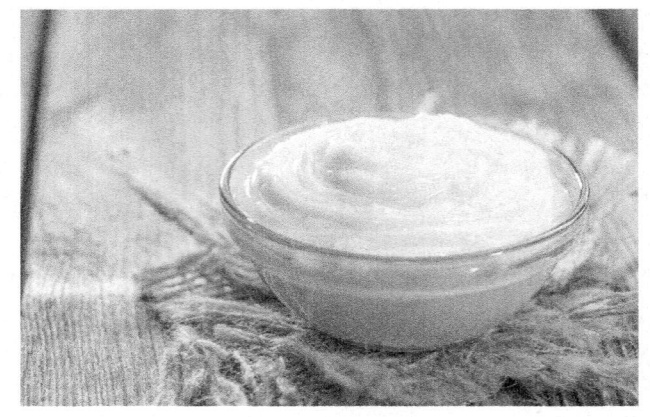

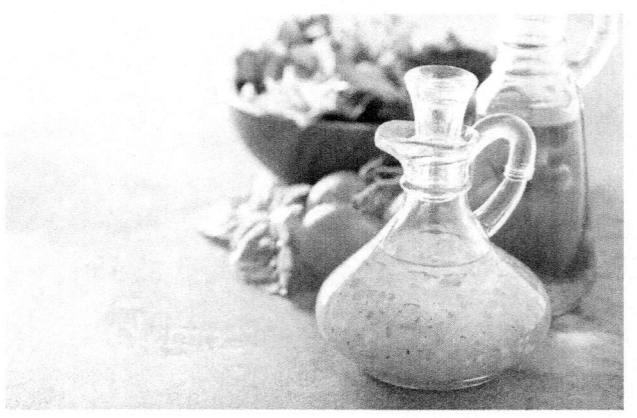

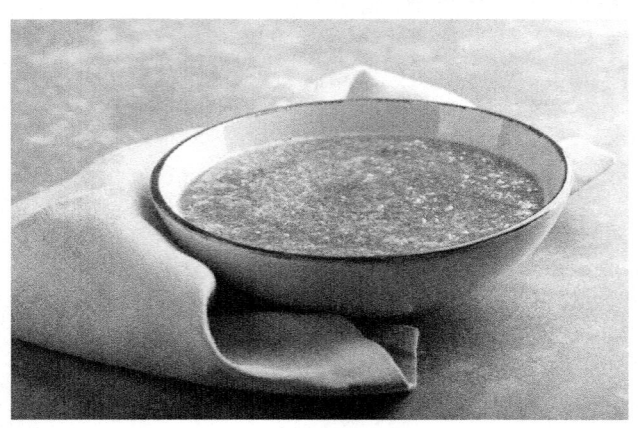

ORANGE-GINGER SAUCE

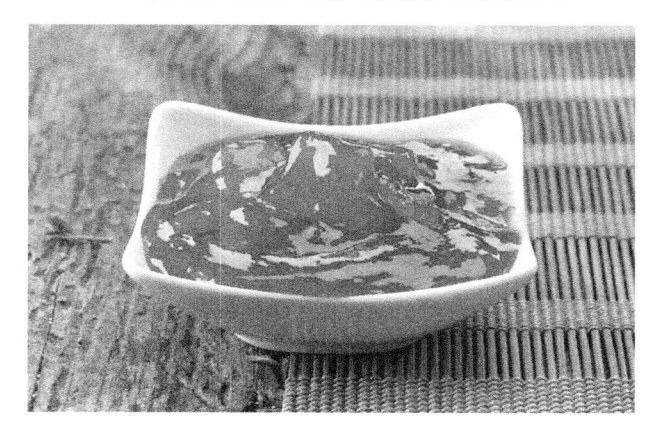

Cooking Time: 35 Minutes
Serving Size: 1/2 Cup

Ingredients
- 1 cup of fresh Orange Juice
- 2 tablespoons of Agave Syrup*
- 1 tablespoon of minced Ginger
- 1 tablespoon of Red Bell Pepper
- 1 tablespoon of Red Onions
- 1/2 teaspoon of crushed Red Pepper**

Cooking Instructions
1. Take a small saucepan. Add all above-mentioned ingredients to it and whisk together.
2. Bring it to a boil on high heat, reduce to a simmer for 12–15 minutes. Whisk the mixture every 2–3 minutes.
3. Pour cooked sauce into a bowl. Let it cool for 12–15 minutes to receive thicker consistency.
4. Serve and enjoy your Orange-Ginger Sauce!

Useful Tips
* If Oranges aren't sweet, add extra tablespoons of Agave Syrup.

SPICY TOMATO SAUCE

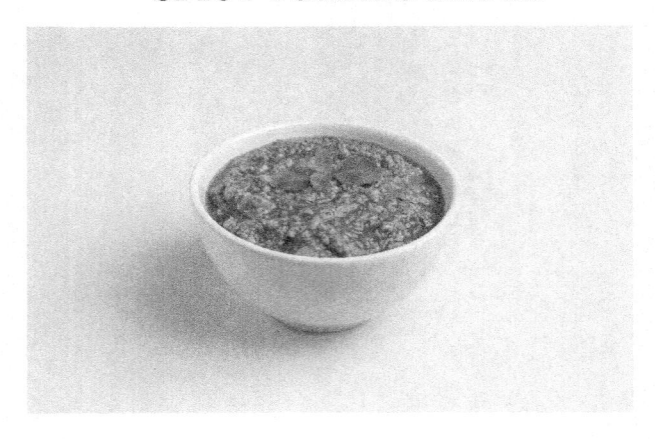

Cooking Time: 2 Hours 10 Minutes
Serving Size: 6 Cups

Ingredients
- 20 Plum Tomatoes
- 2 tablespoons of chopped White Onion
- 2 tablespoons of chopped Red Onion
- 2 tablespoons of chopped Green Bell Pepper
- 2 tablespoons of Agave Syrup
- 2 tablespoons of Oregano
- 2 tablespoons of Basil
- 2 tablespoons of Pure Sea Salt
- 2 tablespoons of Grapeseed Oil
- 1 teaspoon of Cayenne Powder*
- 2 Bay Leaves

Cooking Instructions
1. Boil water in a small pot. Take it away from the heat.
2. Make X-shape cuts on the end of every Plum Tomato. Put them in the pot with hot water for 1 minute.
3. Take the Plum Tomatoes out and shock them with ice-cold water for 30 seconds. Remove the skin easily.

4. Put Plum Tomatoes, Grapeseed Oil, Agave Syrup, and seasonings* in a blender or a food processor. Blend the mixture for 30–40 seconds until it's a smooth consistency.
5. Pour the mixture in a small pot and add 2 Bay Leaves. Simmer the Tomato Sauce on a low heat for about 2 hours.
6. Put chopped Peppers, Onions, and some Grapeseed Oil to a pan. Sauté them for 5 minutes, then add to the sauce.
7. Remove the Bay Leaves before serving.
8. Serve and enjoy your Spicy Tomato Sauce!

Useful Tips

* If you don't want to receive too spicy sauce, add just 1/4 teaspoon of Cayenne Powder.

You can use this Spicy Tomato Sauce within 1 week. Store it in a glass jar with a lid in the refrigerator.

HEMPSEED MAYONNAISE

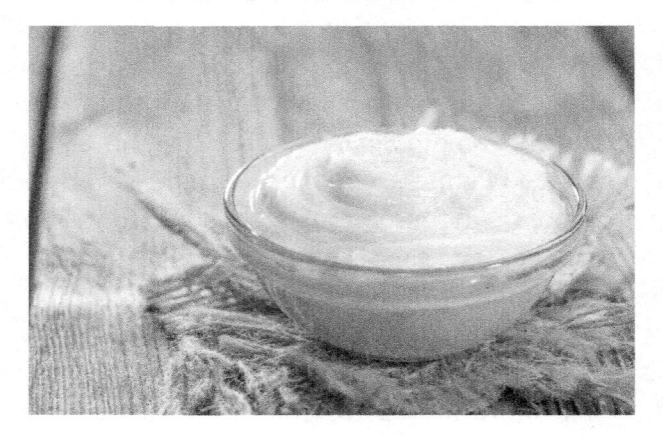

Cooking Time: 5 Minutes
Serving Size: 1–1/2 Cups

Ingredients

- 1 cup of Hemp Seeds
- 2 tablespoons of Grapeseed Oil
- 1 teaspoon of Lime Juice
- 1 tablespoon of Onion Powder
- 1/2 teaspoon of Pure Sea Salt
- 3/4 cup of Spring Water

Cooking Instructions

1. Add all above-mentioned ingredients to a hand blender. Blend well for 40–60 seconds until you reach a smooth consistency.
2. If the mixture is too thick, add more Spring Water. If there is too much liquid, add more Hemp Seeds.
3. Pour it in a jar with a lid and store in the refrigerator.
4. Serve and enjoy your Hempseed Mayonnaise!

TOMATO PIZZA SAUCE

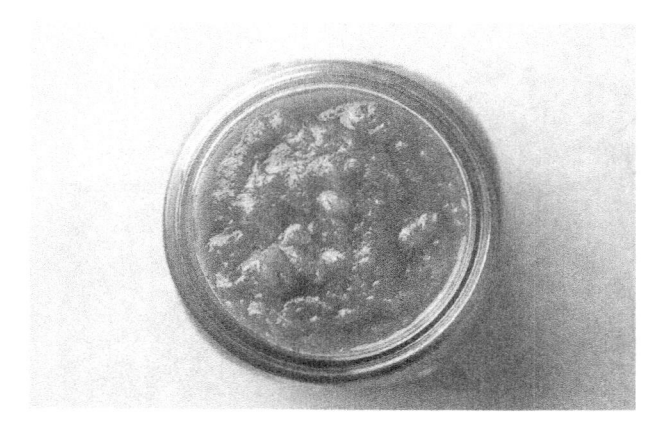

Cooking Time: 10 Minutes
Serving Size: 1–1-1/2 Cups

Ingredients
- 5 Plum Tomatoes
- 2 tablespoons of Agave Syrup
- 2 tablespoons of chopped Onion
- 2 tablespoons of Grapeseed Oil
- 1 teaspoon of Oregano
- 1 teaspoon of Onion Powder
- 1 teaspoon of Pure Sea Salt

Cooking Instructions
1. Boil water in a small pot. Take it away from the heat.
2. Make X-shape cuts on the end of every Plum Tomato. Put them in the pot with hot water for 1 minute. Take the Plum Tomatoes out and shock them with ice-cold water for 30 seconds. Remove the skin easily.
3. Put all prepared ingredients, including Tomatoes, in a blender or food processor. Blend the mixture for 30 seconds until a smooth consistency is reached. Serve and enjoy it!

CHEESE SAUCE

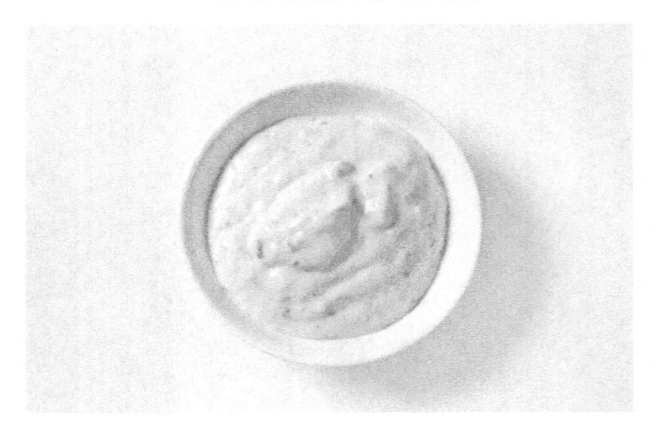

Cooking Time: 3 Hours 15 Minutes
Serving Size: 6 Cups

Ingredients

- 2 cups of raw Brazil Nuts
- 1-1/2 cups *Homemade Hempseed Milk (see recipe on page 114)*
- 1-1/2 cups of Spring Water
- 2 tablespoons of Grapeseed Oil
- 2 teaspoons of Pure Sea Salt
- 1 teaspoon of Onion Powder
- 1/2 teaspoon of Cayenne Powder
- Juice from half of a Lime

Cooking Instructions

1. Soak the raw Brazil Nuts overnight or for at least 3–4 hours. Pour out the water and rinse them thoroughly.
2. Place all ingredients with only 1/2 cup of the Spring Water into a food processor or a blender.
3. Blend all together for about 2–3 minutes.
4. Add another 1/2 cup of the Spring Water and blend it one more time.

5. Continue to add more water if needed. Blend the mixture until it attains a creamy consistency.
6. Allow to cool the sauce mixture before serving.
7. Serve and enjoy your homemade "Cheese" Sauce!

GARLIC SAUCE

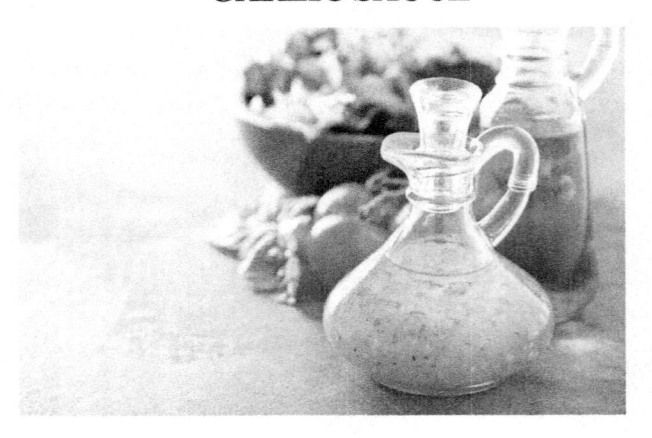

Cooking Time: 1 Hour 10 Minutes
Serving Size: 1 Cup

Ingredients
- 1 tablespoon of Onion Powder
- 1/2 teaspoon of Ginger
- 1/4 cup of diced Shallots
- 1/4 teaspoon of Dill
- 1 cup of Grapeseed Oil
- 1/2 teaspoon of Pure Sea Salt

Cooking Instructions
1. Get a glass jar with a lid. Put all above-mentioned ingredients in the jar. Shake them well until smooth.
2. Place the jar with sauce mixture in the refrigerator for at least 1 hour. Serve and enjoy your "Garlic" Sauce!

Useful Tips
You can use this "Garlic" Sauce within 2 weeks. Store it in a glass jar with a lid in the refrigerator.
If you have a hand blender, mix all ingredients together. The sauce is prepared and you can use it immediately.

SALSA VERDE

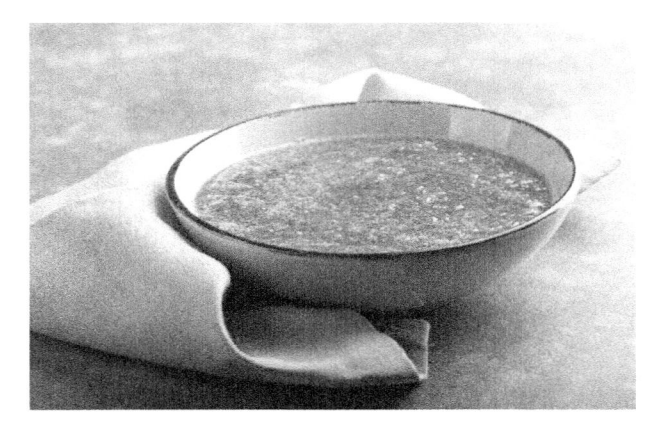

Cooking Time: 25 Minutes
Serving Size: 2 Cups

Ingredients

- 1 pound of Tomatillos
- 1/2 cup of chopped Onions
- 1/4 cup of fresh Cilantro
- 1 teaspoon of Oregano
- 1 teaspoon of Onion Powder
- 1 teaspoon of Pure Sea Salt

Cooking Instructions

1. Remove the skin from Tomatillos. Rinse them and cut in half.
2. Put all ingredients (except Cilantro) in a medium saucepan and add Spring Water to cover Tomatillos.
3. Bring to a boil and cook on medium heat for 15–20 minutes. Stir occasionally.
4. Strain the ingredients, add them to a blender with Cilantro, and blend for 30–40 seconds.
5. Serve and enjoy your Salsa Verde!

WHITE QUESO DIP

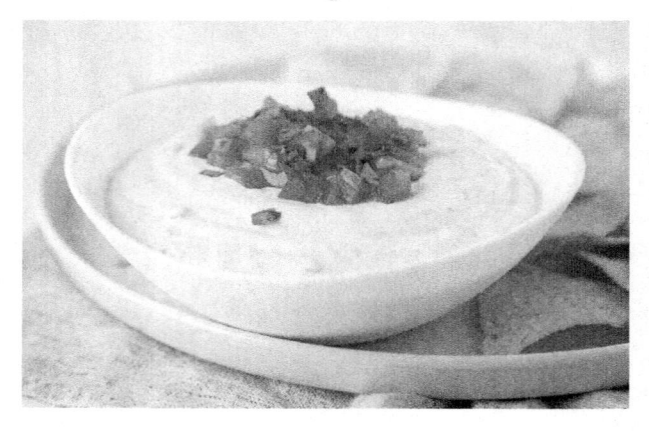

Cooking Time: 10 Minutes
Serving Size: 2 Cups

Ingredients

- 1 cup of soaked Brazil Nuts (overnight or at least 3 hours)
- 1/4 cup of diced White and Red Onions
- 1/4 cup of diced Green and Red Bell Peppers
- 1/2 cup + 2 tablespoons *of Homemade Hempseed Milk (see recipe on page 114)*
- 1 tablespoon of Sea Moss Gel*
- 1/2 teaspoon of Pure Sea Salt
- 1 teaspoon of Onion Powder
- 1 teaspoon of Grapeseed Oil
- 1/4 teaspoon of Cayenne Powder**
- 1/4 cup of Spring Water

Cooking Instructions

1. Put soaked Brazil Nuts, Spring Water, Sea Moss Gel*, and seasonings** in a blender. Blend ingredients well until smooth.
2. Take a small saucepan, add Grapeseed Oil, Onions, and Peppers. Lightly sauté on medium heat for 2 minutes.

3. Pour the blended mixture in the saucepan. If it is too thick, add extra Spring Water.
4. Cook on low heat for 2–3 minutes.
5. Serve and enjoy your White Queso Dip!

Useful Tips

* Adding Sea Moss Gel helps to make a smoother consistency. But if you don't have it, you can skip it.

** If you like spicy sauces, you can add 1/2 teaspoon of Cayenne Powder instead.

SPECIAL INGREDIENTS

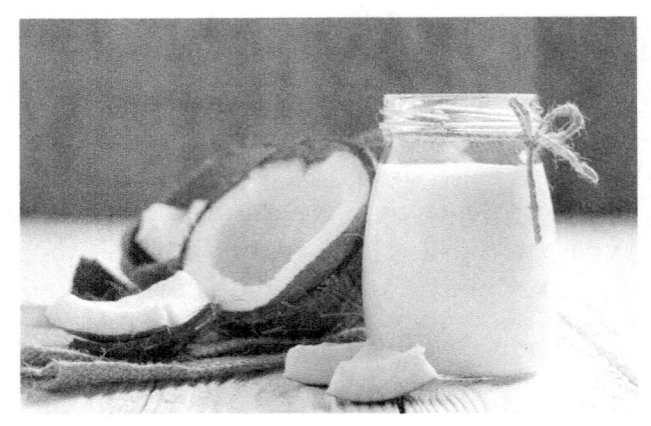

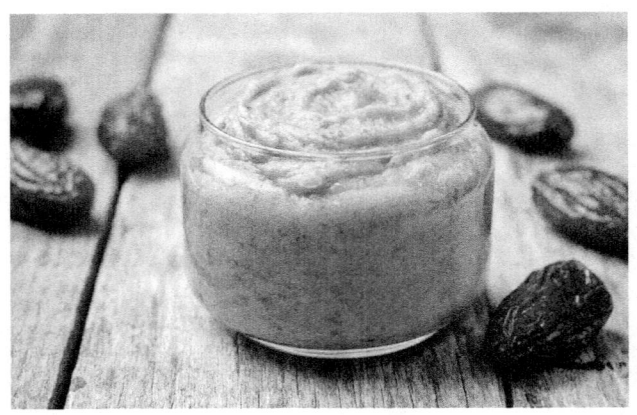

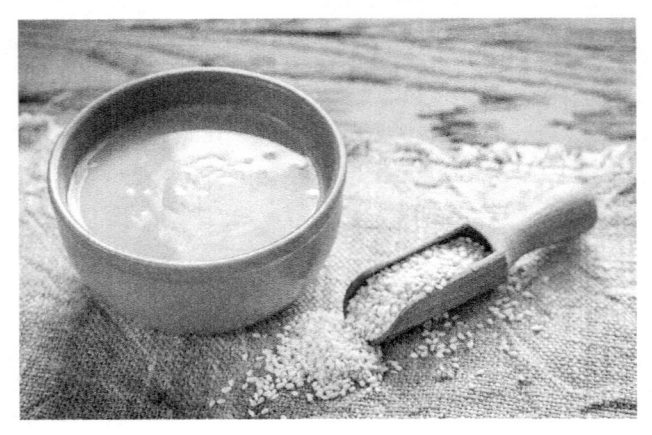

HOMEMADE WALNUT MILK

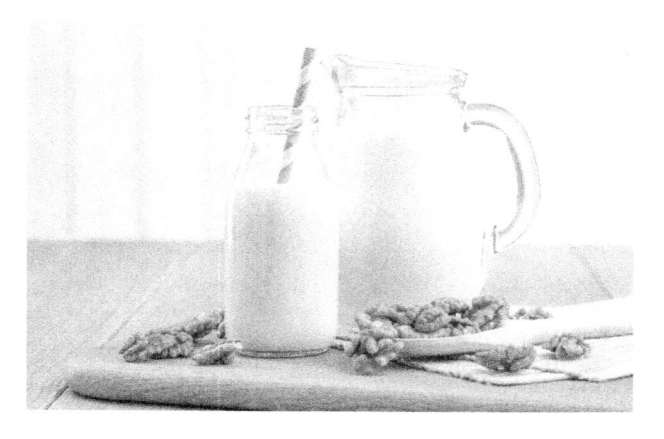

Cooking Time: Minimum 8 Hours
Serving Size: 4 Cups

Ingredients

- 1 cup raw Walnuts
- 3 cups of Spring Water + extra for soaking
- 1/8 teaspoon of Pure Sea Salt

Cooking Instructions

1. Place the raw Walnuts in a medium bowl and cover them with 3 inches of water.
2. Leave the Walnuts in the water for at least 8 hours or overnight.
3. Drain them and rinse with cold water.
4. Add the soaked Walnuts, 3 cups of Spring Water, and Pure Sea Salt in a blender.
5. Mix all ingredients well until smooth.
6. Strain it if you need to.
7. Enjoy your Homemade Walnut Milk!

AQUAFABA

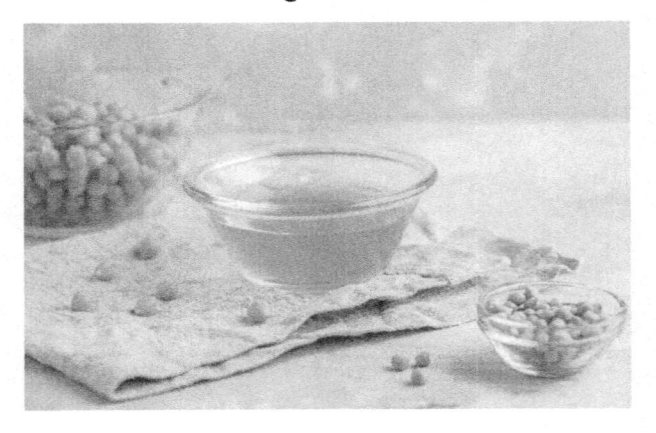

Cooking Time: 2 Hours 30 Minutes
Serving Size: 2–4 Cups

Ingredients
- 1 bag of Garbanzo Beans
- 6 cups of Spring Water + extra for soaking
- 1 teaspoon of Pure Sea Salt

Cooking Instructions
1. Add Garbanzo Beans, Spring Water, and Pure Sea Salt in a large pot.
2. Bring it to a rolling boil.
3. Remove from the heat and leave to soak for 30–40 minutes.
4. Strain Garbanzo Beans and add 6 cups of fresh Spring Water.
5. Bring it to a rolling boil.
6. Reduce to medium heat.
7. Simmer the mixture repeatedly for 1 hour and 30 minutes on medium heat.
8. Strain the Garbanzo Beans. This strained water is Aquafaba.

9. Pour Aquafaba into a glass jar with a lid and place it in the refrigerator.
10. After cooling, Aquafaba becomes thicker.
11. If there is too much liquid, repeatedly boil for 10–20 minutes.

Useful Tips

Aquafaba is a good alternative for an egg:
- 2 tablespoons of Aquafaba = 1 egg white
- 3 tablespoons of Aquafaba = 1 egg.

Aquafaba can be kept in the refrigerator for up to 5 days. Store it in a glass jar with a lid.

HOMEMADE COCONUT MILK

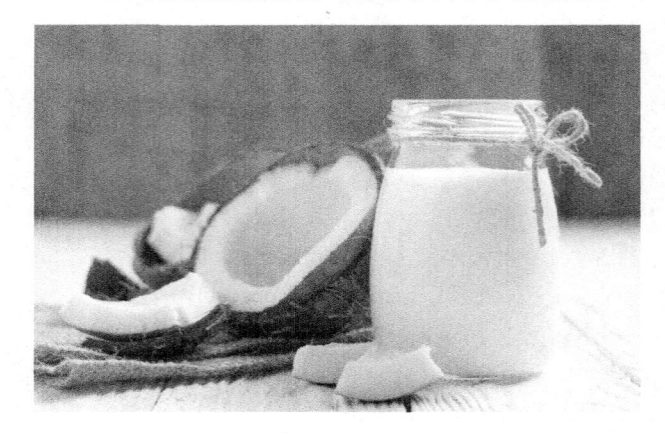

Cooking Time: 10 Minutes
Serving Size: Varies (depending on the size of coconut)*

Ingredients
- 1 young Coconut.
- 1/4 cup of Spring Water
- Agave Syrup, to taste

Cooking Instructions
1. Put the Coconut on one side. Cut the husk off slice by slice until you reach the brown part.
2. Cut a big triangle on the brown top of the Coconut. Remove this part from the Coconut. You should see a triangle hole on the top of it.
3. Pour coconut water in a blender.
4. Scoop out coconut meat with a spoon and put it in the blender.
5. Blend it for 2 minutes until mixed well.
6. Strain the mixture through a nut milk bag and add Agave Syrup, to taste.
7. If the milk consistency is too thick, add Spring Water and blend it repeatedly.
8. Enjoy your Homemade Coconut Milk!

HOMEMADE TAHINI BUTTER

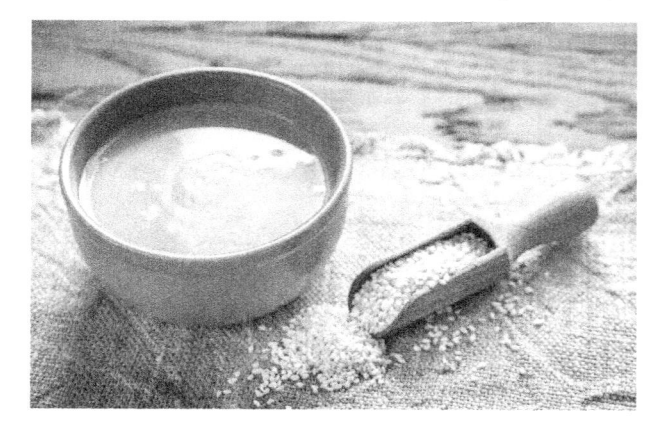

Cooking Time: 5 Minutes
Serving Size: 1 Cup

Ingredients
- 1 cup of raw Sesame Seeds
- 1–2 tablespoons of Grapeseed Oil

Cooking Instructions
1. Put raw Sesame Seeds in a blender.
2. Blend well until it becomes chunky.
3. Add Grapeseed Oil to the mixture*.
4. Mix until smooth consistency.
5. Put the butter in a glass jar with a lid**.
6. Serve and enjoy your Homemade Tahini Butter!

Useful Tips
* You can add some Pure Sea Salt or Agave Syrup, to taste.
** If you don't use it at once, store the Tahini Butter in a refrigerator.

HOMEMADE DATE SUGAR

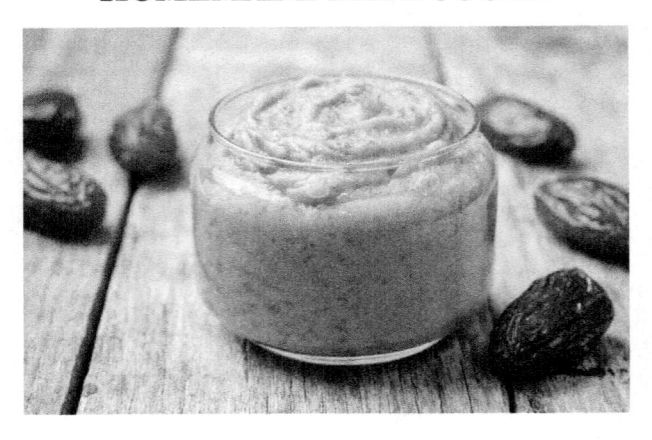

Cooking Time: 25 Minutes
Serving Size: 1-1/2 Cups

Ingredients
- 1 cup of Dates

Cooking Instructions
1. Preheat your oven to 400°F.
2. Divide the Dates in half. Remove all the seeds from them*.
3. Take a baking pan and cover it with a piece of parchment paper. Put all the halves on the paper.
4. Bake for about 12–15 minutes**. The Dates can become slightly burnt. Take them out and let cool.
5. After they have cooled, the Dates should become hard like candies. If they are not so hard, bake for more 3–5 more minutes.
6. Grind the baked halves in a blender for 20 seconds.
7. Enjoy your Homemade Date Sugar!

Useful Tips
* If you wish, you can use Dates without the seeds.
** If the Dates are large, it might require an extra 3–5 minutes for baking.

HOMEMADE DATE SYRUP

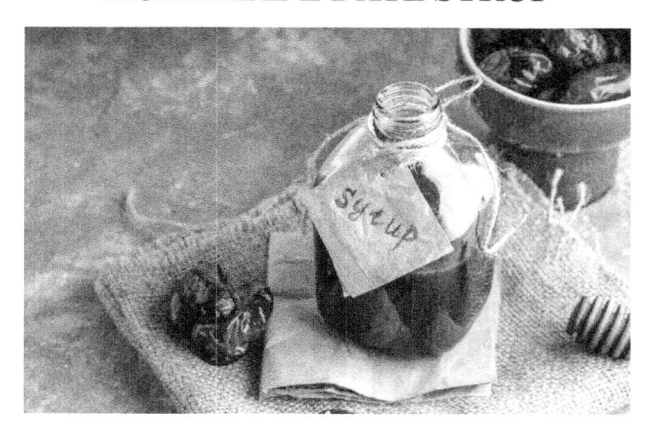

Cooking Time: 20 Minutes
Serving Size: 2–2-1/2 Cups

Ingredients
- 1 cup of Dates
- 1 cup of Spring Water

Cooking Instructions
1. Pour water in a small pot and heat it up on the stovetop. Remove from the heat.
2. Place the Dates in the warm water and leave there for 15 minutes.
3. Pour Spring Water with Dates into a blender. Blend them well until achieving smooth consistency.
4. If it is too thick, add extra Spring Water (about 1/4 cup) and blend repeatedly.
5. Pour in a jar with a lid. Store in the refrigerator.
6. Enjoy your Homemade Date Syrup!

Useful Tips
Unlike *Homemade Date Sugar (see recipe on page 112)*, this Homemade Date Syrup can be dissolved in tea.

HOMEMADE HEMPSEED MILK

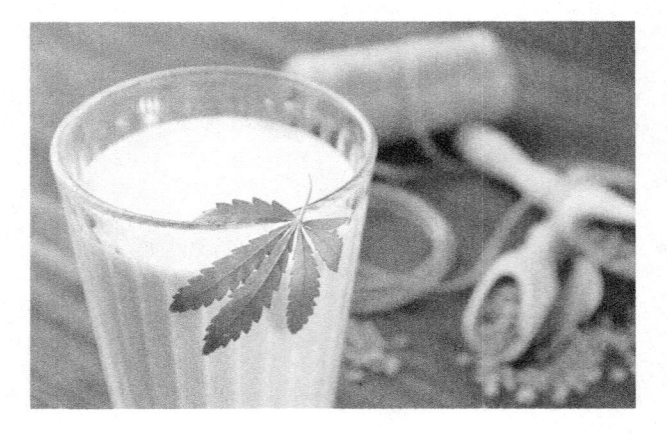

Cooking Time: 2 Hours
Serving Size: 2 Cups

Ingredients

- 2 cups of Spring Water
- 2 tablespoons of Agave Syrup
- 2 tablespoons of Hemp Seeds
- 1/8 teaspoon of Pure Sea Salt
- Fruits (optional)*

Cooking Instructions

1. Place all above-mentioned ingredients (except fruits) into a blender. Blend them well for 2 minutes.
2. Add fruits* (if you want) and repeatedly blend for 1 minute.
3. Pour milk into a glass jar with a lid. Leave it in a refrigerator until cold. Enjoy your Homemade Hempseed Milk!

Useful Tips

* You can add Baby Bananas, or any other fruits from *Dr. Sebi's approved food list (check it on page 22)* to the milk.

It can be kept in the refrigerator for up to 5 days. However, if you add fruits to the milk, it will only be fresh for 24 hours.

SNACKS & BREAD

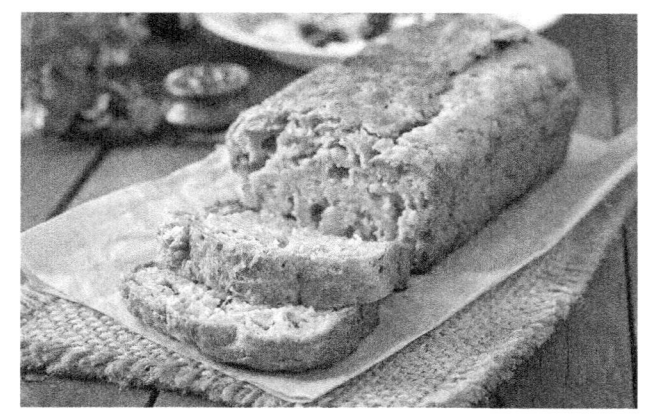

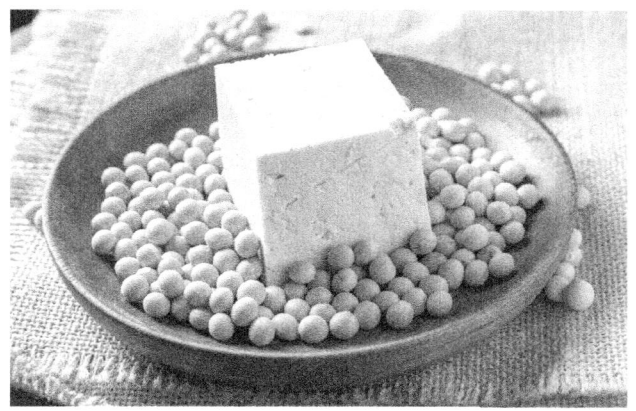

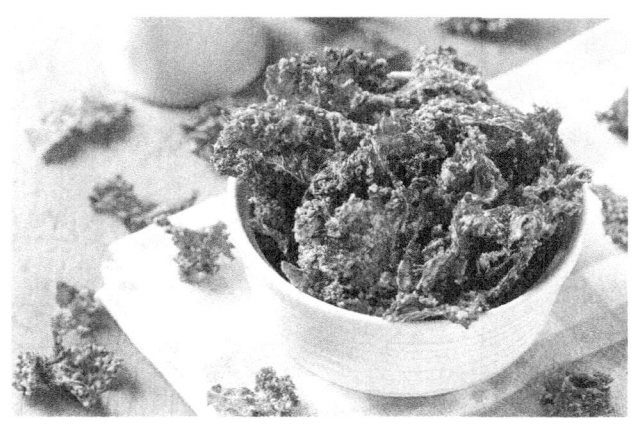

TORTILLAS

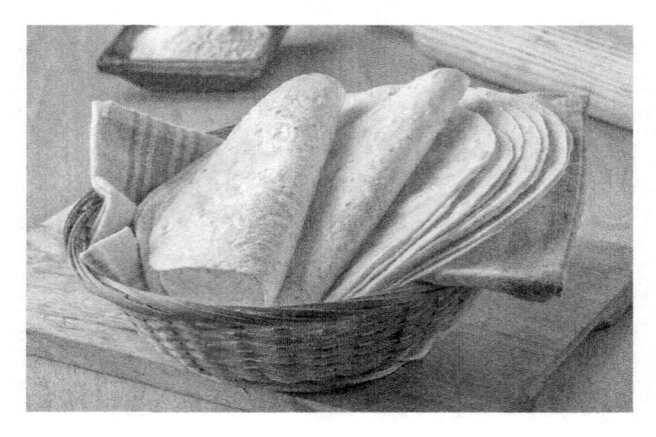

Cooking Time: 20 Minutes
Serving Size: 8 Servings

Ingredients

- 2 cups of Spelt Flour
- 1/2 cup of Spring Water
- 1 teaspoon of Pure Sea Salt

Cooking Instructions

1. Pour out the Spelt Flour with Pure Sea Salt in a food processor*. Mix them for 15 seconds.
2. Continue to blend while slowly adding Grapeseed Oil until well incorporated.
3. Slowly add Spring Water while blending until a dough is formed.
4. Prepare a work surface for kneading. Cover it with a piece of parchment paper and sprinkle with flour.
5. Knead the dough until the ball is formed. Divide the formed dough into 8 equal balls.
6. Roll out each ball into a very thin circle.
7. Take a non-stick pan and warm it on high heat.
8. Place one dough circle on the pan. Cook one tortilla at a time on medium heat for 30–60 seconds on each side.

9. Serve** and enjoy your Tortillas!

Useful Tips

* If you don't have a food processor, you can substitute it with a blender or a hand mixer. However, you will achieve better results using a food processor.

** You can serve cooked Tortillas with our *"Cheese" Sauce (see recipe on page 100), Spicy Tomato Sauce (see recipe on page 96), Orange-Ginger Sauce (see recipe on page 95), Salsa Verde (see recipe on page 103),* or *White Queso Dip (see recipe on page 104).*

TORTILLA CHIPS

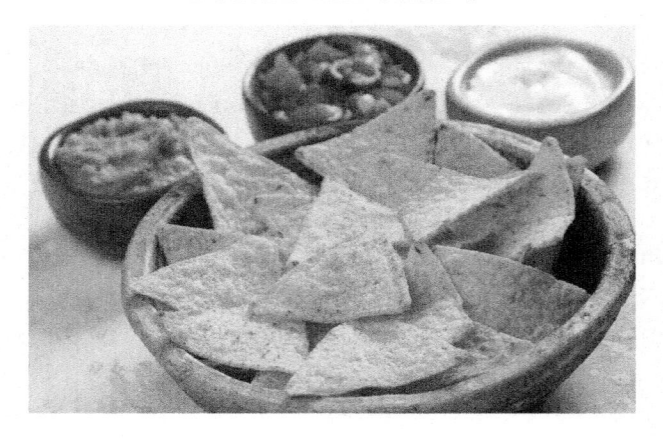

Cooking Time: 30 Minutes
Serving Size: 8 Servings

Ingredients
- 2 cups of Spelt Flour
- 1/2 cup of Spring Water
- 1/3 cup of Grapeseed Oil
- 1 teaspoon of Pure Sea Salt

Cooking Instructions
1. Preheat your oven to 350°F.
2. Pour out the Spelt Flour with Pure Sea Salt in a food processor*. Mix them for 15 seconds.
3. Continue to blend while slowly adding Grapeseed Oil until well incorporated.
4. Slowly add Spring Water while blending until a dough is formed.
5. Prepare a work surface for kneading. Cover it with a piece of parchment paper and sprinkle with flour.
6. Knead the dough until the ball is formed.
7. Divide the formed dough into 8 equal balls.
8. Roll out each ball into a very thin circle.
9. Cover a baking pan with a little Grapeseed Oil.

10. Put the rolled out dough on the baking pan.
11. Brush dough with a little Grapeseed Oil and sprinkle with Pure Sea Salt if desired.
12. Using a pizza slicer cut the dough into 6–8 triangles.
13. Bake for about 10–12 minutes or until the chips are starting to become golden-brown.
14. Allow to cool before serving.
15. Serve** and enjoy your Tortilla Chips!

Useful Tips

* If you don't have a food processor, you can substitute it with a blender or a hand mixer. However, you will achieve better results using a food processor.

** You can serve cooked Tortillas Chips with our *"Cheese" Sauce (see recipe on page 100)*, *Spicy Tomato Sauce (see recipe on page 96)*, *Orange-Ginger Sauce (see recipe on page 95)*, *Salsa Verde (see recipe on page 103)*, or *White Queso Dip (see recipe on page 104)*.

HERB BREAD

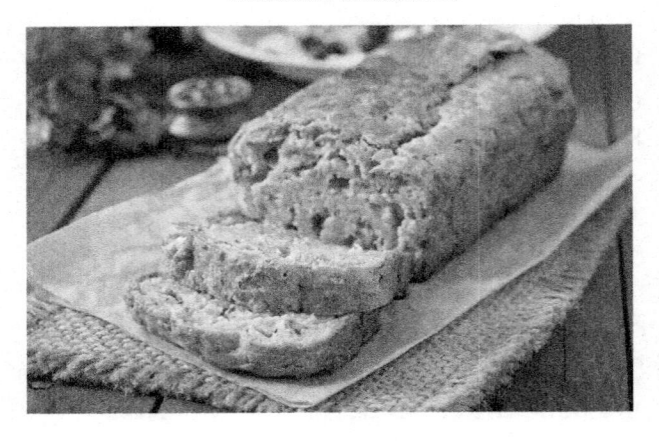

Cooking Time: 1 Hour
Serving Size: 1 Loaf

Ingredients

- 4 cups of Chickpea Flour
- 1/2 cup of *Homemade Date Syrup (see recipe on page 113)*
- 1-1/2 cups of Spring Water
- 3 tablespoons of Grapeseed Oil
- 1 tablespoon of Onion Powder
- 1 tablespoon of Pure Sea Salt
- 1 teaspoon of Thyme
- 1 teaspoon of Oregano
- 1 teaspoon of Basil

Cooking Instructions

1. Preheat your oven to 350°F.
2. Put all dry ingredients in a mixing bowl and blend them.
3. Add Oil, Date Syrup, and 1 cup of Spring Water. Stir gently.
4. Pour the prepared mixture into a loaf pan. Coat with some Grapeseed Oil and sprinkle top with extra herbs.
5. Bake for 50–60 minutes. Let it cool before cutting.
6. Serve and enjoy your Herb Bread!

CHICKPEA "TOFU"

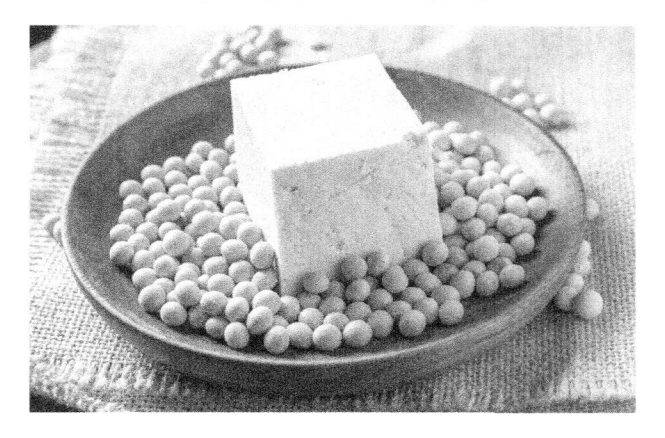

Cooking Time: 40 Minutes
Serving Size: 2–4 Servings

Ingredients
- 1 cup of Chickpea Flour
- 2 cups of Spring Water
- 1 teaspoon of Parsley
- 1 teaspoon of Pure Sea Salt

Cooking Instructions
1. Cover a baking dish with a piece of parchment paper.
2. Add all ingredients in a saucepan, whisk them together on medium heat.
3. Continue whisking for 3–5 minutes until it becomes thicker.
4. Pour "tofu" batter into the baking dish and spread it with a spoon.
5. Let it cool for 30 minutes until firm; placing it in the refrigerator will speed it up.
6. Take it out and cut into medium cubes.
7. Serve and enjoy your Chickpea "Tofu"!

KALE CHIPS

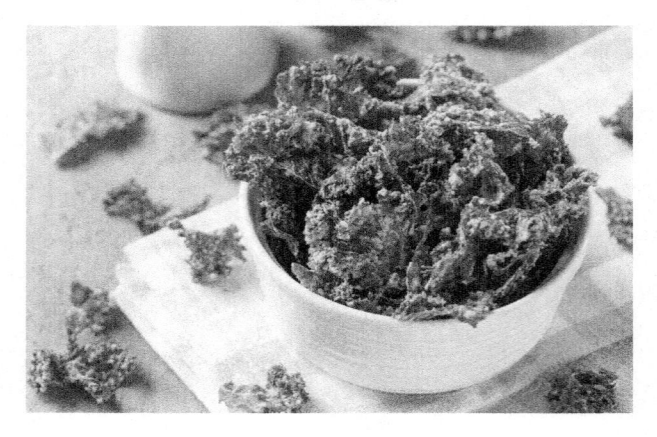

Cooking Time: 20 Minutes
Serving Size: 2–4 Servings

Ingredients

- 1 pound of Kale
- 2 teaspoons of Grapeseed Oil
- Pure Sea Salt, to taste
- Onion Powder, to taste
- Cayenne Powder, to taste

Cooking Instructions

1. Preheat your oven to 350°F.
2. Rinse off the Kale and dry with paper towels.
3. Cut the Kale leaves near the stem using scissors. Make sure not to cut them too small.
4. Place the leaves in a bowl, add seasonings, and sprinkle with Grapeseed Oil. Mix it.
5. Take a baking pan and cover it with a piece of parchment paper. Put the Kale leaves on it and bake them in the oven for 7–8 minutes.
6. Repeat the last step until all Kale leaves are cooked.
7. Serve and enjoy your Kale Chips!

DESSERTS

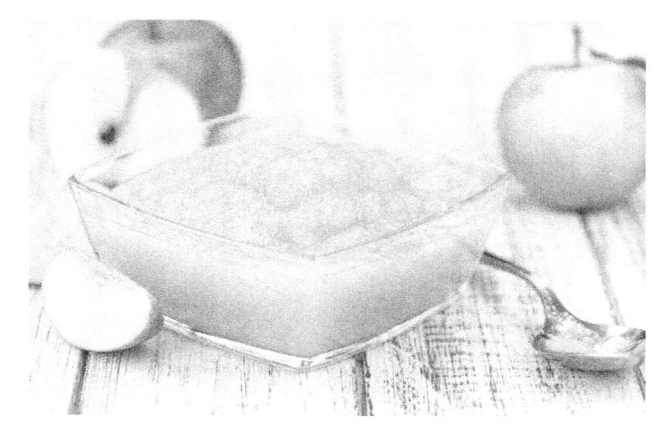

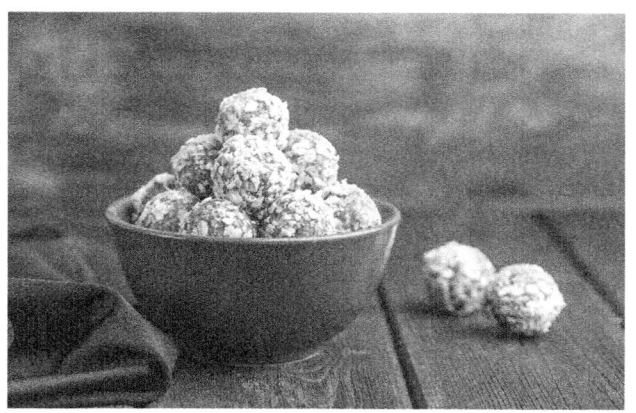

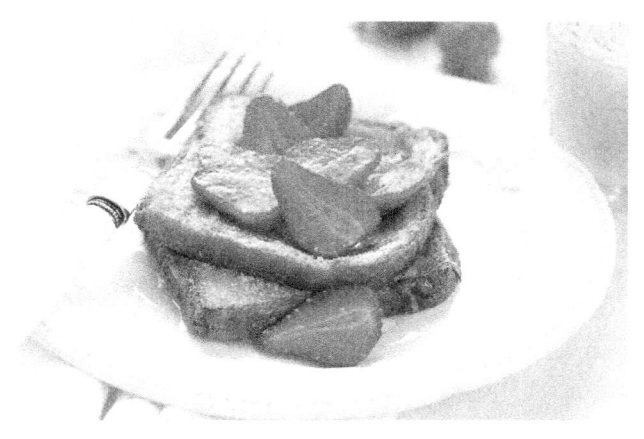

BANANA PIE

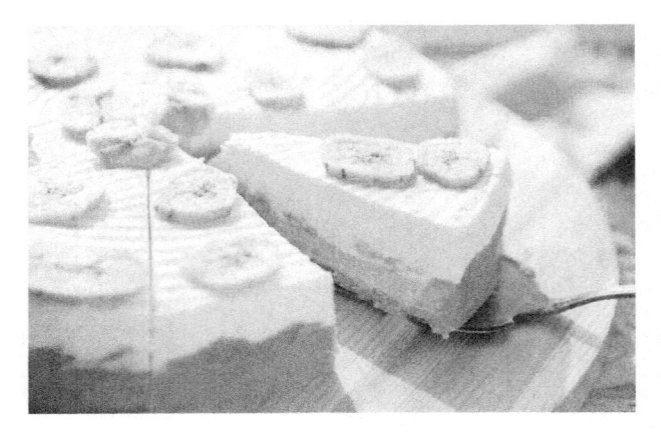

Cooking Time: 40 Minutes + 4 Hours in the freezer
Serving Size: 6–8 Servings

Ingredients
Crust
- 1-1/2 cups of pitted Dates
- 1-1/2 cups of shredded Soft-Jelly Coconut
- 1/4 cup of Agave Syrup
- 1/4 teaspoon of Pure Sea Salt

Filling
- 6–8 Burro Bananas
- 1 cup of *Homemade Hempseed Milk (see recipe on page 114)**
- 7 ounces of Organic Creamed Unsweetened Coconut
- 4 tablespoons of Agave Syrup
- 1/8 teaspoon of Pure Sea Salt

Cooking Instructions
1. Add crust ingredients in a blender.
2. Blend them for about 30 seconds or until the ball is formed.

3. Cover the round pie pan with parchment paper, put crust mixture inside, and spread it out.
4. Store it in the refrigerator for about 10 minutes to firm up the crust.
5. Put all filling ingredients in a large bowl and mix them until well combined.
6. Pour the filling into a pan and spread it by shaking the sides.
7. Cover the pie with foil and put it in the freezer for about 4 hours to firm up.
8. Serve with some banana slides on the top.
9. Enjoy your Banana Pie!

Useful Tips

* If you don't have *Homemade Hempseed Milk*, you can substitute it with *Homemade Walnut Milk (see recipe on page 107)*.

MANGO CHEESECAKE

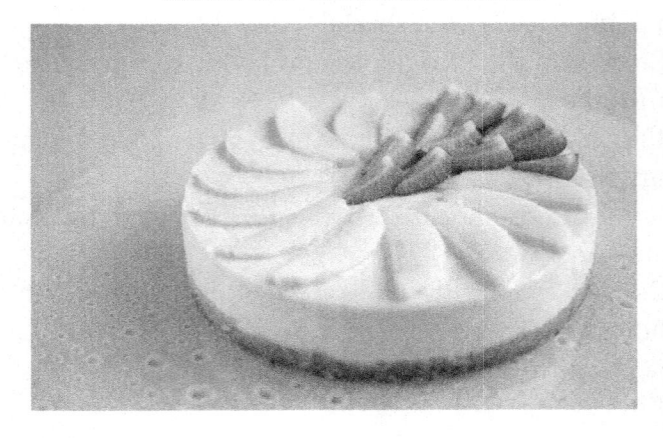

Cooking Time: 30 Minutes + 2–4 Hours in the refrigerator
Serving Size: 6–8 Servings

Ingredients
<u>Crust</u>
- 1 cup of Walnuts
- 1 cup of Dates
- 1/4 cup of shredded Soft-Jelly Coconut

<u>Filling</u>
- 2 chopped large Mangoes
- 2 cups of soaked Walnuts (overnight or at least 4 hours)
- 1 cup of *Homemade Coconut Milk (see recipe on page 110)*
- 1/3 cup of Agave Syrup
- 6 tablespoons of Coconut Oil
- 1 tablespoon of Key Lime Zest
- Juice of 1 Key Lime

Cooking Instructions
1. Take an 8-inch round cake pan and cover it with a piece of parchment paper.

2. Put Walnuts, shredded Soft-Jelly Coconut, and Dates in a food processor or a blender. Mix it until well combined. Add more Dates, if the dough is not sticky.
3. Put the prepared dough into the pan, press and spread it. Place it in the freezer for 10 minutes.
4. Add Coconut Milk with Walnuts into a blender or a food processor and blend it for 2–3 minutes until a smooth consistency. Add Agave Syrup, chopped Mango, Coconut Oil, Key Lime Zest, and Juice. Continue mixing until well combined.
5. Pour the cheesecake filling into the pan and spread it.
6. Place prepared cheesecake in the freezer for 2–4 hours until it firms up.
7. Serve and enjoy your Mango Cheesecake!

COCONUT WAFFLE

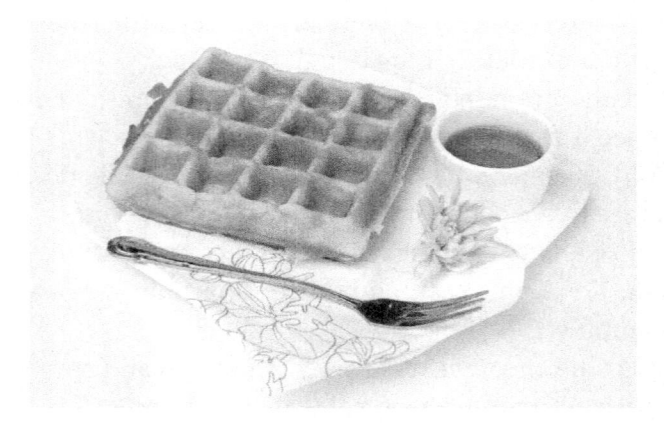

Cooking Time: 20 Minutes
Serving Size: 1 Serving

Ingredients

- 2 cups of Spelt Flour
- 1 cup of *Homemade Coconut Milk (see recipe on page 110)*
- 1/4 cup of Coconut Flour
- 1/4 cup of Agave Syrup
- 2 teaspoons of Sea Moss Gel
- 1/4 teaspoon of Pure Sea Salt
- 3 tablespoons of Grapeseed Oil
- 1 cup of Spring Water

Cooking Instructions

1. Add Spelt Flour, Coconut Flour, and Pure Sea Salt in a bowl and blend them.
2. Mix together *Homemade Coconut Milk,* Sea Moss Gel, Agave Syrup, Grapeseed Oil, and Spring Water in a separate bowl. Pour the liquid mixture into the dry mix.
3. Pour the prepared batter into a waffle maker and cook following its instructions.
4. Serve with Agave Syrup and enjoy your Coconut Waffles!

APPLESAUCE

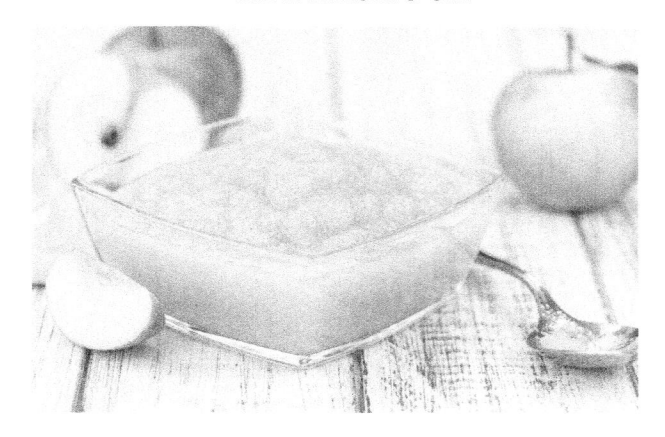

Cooking Time: 15 Minutes
Serving Size: 4 Servings

Ingredients

- 3 cups of chopped Apples
- 1/2 cup of Strawberries *(or any other fruits from Dr. Sebi Food list)*
- 3 tablespoons of Agave Syrup
- 1 teaspoon of Sea Moss Gel (optional)
- 1 teaspoon of Key Lime Juice
- 1/8 teaspoon of Pure Sea Salt
- 1/8 teaspoon of Cloves
- 1 tablespoon of Spring Water, if needed

Cooking Instructions

1. Add chopped Apples, Agave Syrup, Key Lime Juice, Cloves, and Pure Sea Salt into a blender.
2. Mix it well until you reach a smooth consistency.
3. Add Strawberries* in the mixture and continue blending until combined.
4. Pour Spring Water in if the mixture is too thick.
5. Serve and enjoy your Applesauce!

FRENCH TOAST

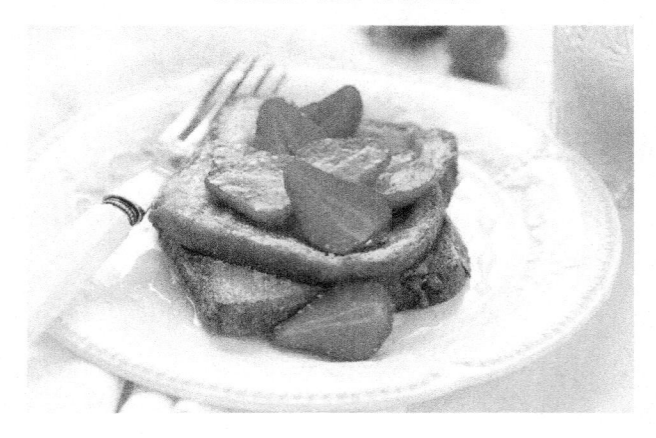

Cooking Time: 25 Minutes
Serving Size: 3–4 Servings

Ingredients

- *Herb Bread (see recipe on page 120)*
- 5–6 sliced Strawberries
- 3/4 cup of *Homemade Hempseed Milk (see recipe on page 114)**
- 1/2 cup of Chickpea Flour
- 2 tablespoons of Agave Syrup
- 1/2 teaspoon of Ground Cloves
- 1/4 teaspoon of Ginger Powder
- 1/4 teaspoon of Pure Sea Salt
- 2 teaspoons of Grapeseed Oil
- 1/4 cup of Spring Water

Cooking Instructions

1. Add *Homemade Hempseed Milk**, Chickpea Flour, Agave Syrup, Spring Water, Ground Cloves, Ginger Powder, and Pure Sea Salt in a large container and mix them together.
2. Cut *Herb Bread* into pieces.

3. Put bread slices in the container and allow to soak for 8–10 minutes, flipping halfway through.
4. Preheat a skillet and lightly grease it with some Grapeseed Oil.
5. Cook every slice of bread on medium heat for 3–4 minutes until golden-brown.
6. Serve with some Agave Syrup and sliced Strawberries on the top.
7. Enjoy your French Toast!

Useful Tips

* If you don't have *Homemade Hempseed Milk*, you can substitute it with *Homemade Walnut Milk (see recipe on page 107)*.

ALKALINE PORRIDGE

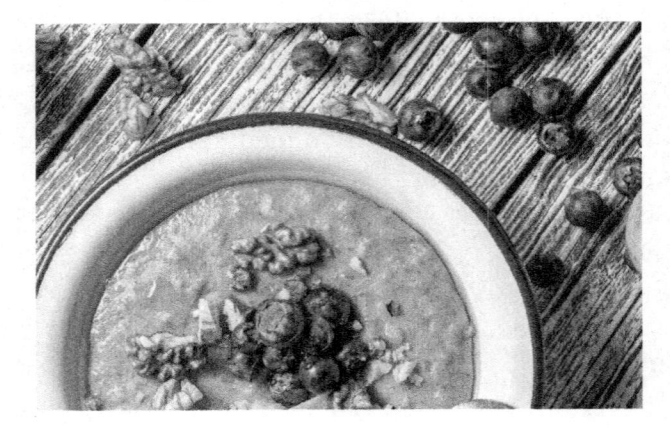

Cooking Time: 25 Minutes
Serving Size: 2–4 Servings

Ingredients

- 1/2 cup of Teff Grain
- Blueberries*
- Walnuts (optional)
- Agave Syrup (optional)
- 2 cups of Spring Water
- Pinch of Pure Sea Salt

Cooking Instructions

1. Pour Spring Water into a small pot and bring it to a boil.
2. Add a pinch of Pure Sea Salt.
3. Put Teff Grain slowly into the boiling water, stirring it.
4. Reduce to low heat, cover with a lid, and simmer for about 15 minutes.
5. Serve with Blueberries*, Walnuts, and some Agave Syrup.
6. Enjoy your Alkaline Porridge!

Useful Tips

* You can add other fruits from *Dr. Sebi's Food List (check it on page 22)* like Strawberries, Pears, or Peaches.

DATE BALLS

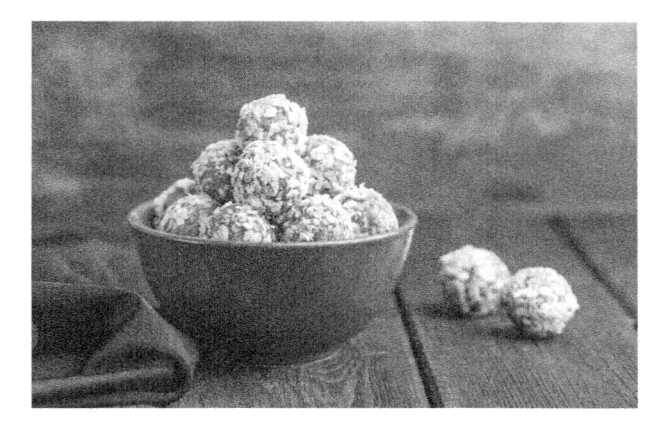

Cooking Time: 30 Minutes
Serving Size: 20–24 Servings

Ingredients
- 1 cup of pitted Dates
- 1 cup of shredded Soft-Jelly Coconut
- 1/2 cup of Sesame Seeds
- 1/2 cup of Brazil Nuts*
- 1/4 cup of Agave Syrup
- 1/2 teaspoon of Pure Sea Salt

Cooking Instructions
1. Add Dates, shredded Coconut, Brazil Nuts*, Agave Syrup, and Pure Sea Salt in a food processor or a blender.
2. Blend it well for about 20–30 seconds.
3. Take a spoon of the prepared mixture in your hand and make a ball. Put Sesame Seeds in a large bowl and roll Date Balls in this mixture.
4. Repeat the step 3 until all of the Date mixture is used.
5. Serve and enjoy your Date Balls!

Useful Tips
* If you don't have Brazil Nuts, you can add Walnuts instead.

STRAWBERRY JAM

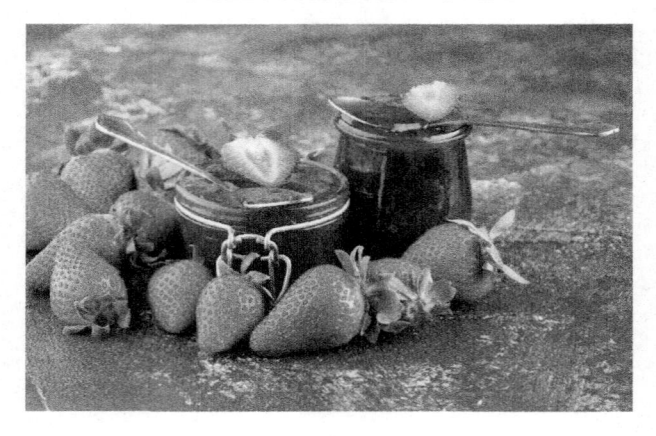

Cooking Time: 30 Minutes
Serving Size: 2 Cups

Ingredients
- 4 cups of chopped Strawberries
- 2/3 cup of Agave Syrup
- 1/2 cup of Sea Moss Gel
- 3 tablespoons of Key Lime Juice

Cooking Instructions
1. Wash and chop all Strawberries into a bowl.
2. Mash them to a chunky consistency.
3. Put Key Lime Juice, Strawberry mixture, and Agave Syrup in a medium saucepan and cook for 10 minutes on medium-high heat, stirring occasionally.
4. Add Sea Moss Gel to a saucepan and cook for 5 more minutes, stirring it to dissolve evenly.
5. Take it away from the heat and allow to cool before using it.
6. Serve and enjoy your Strawberry Jam!

PANCAKES

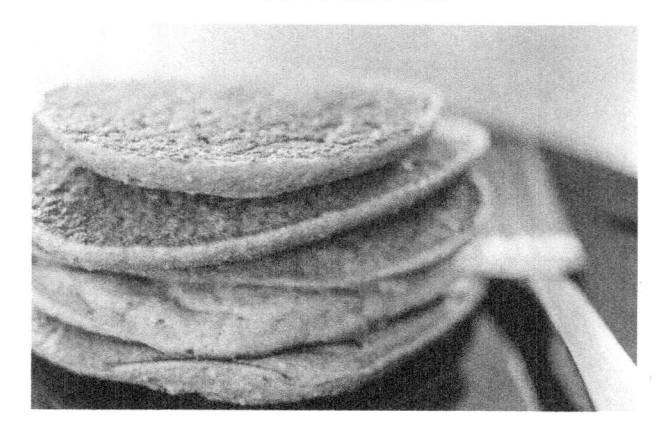

Cooking Time: 30 Minutes
Serving Size: 2 Servings

Ingredients
- 1 cup of Spelt Flour
- 1/2 cup of Blueberries
- 1/4 cup of Agave Syrup
- 1 teaspoon of Vanilla Extract
- 2 pinches of Pure Sea Salt
- 1 teaspoon Grapeseed Oil + more for cooking
- Spring Water (varying on the batter thickness)*

Cooking Instructions
1. Add Spelt Flour, Vanilla Extract, Pure Sea Salt, Spring Water*, and Grapeseed Oil to a bowl and mix them well until combined. Add Blueberries to the mixture and lightly stir.
2. Put a pan on medium heat and lightly grease it with some Grapeseed Oil. Pour part of the batter in the warm pan and cook on both sides until brown.
3. Repeat the step 2 until all Pancakes are cooked.
4. Serve with Agave Syrup and enjoy your Pancakes!

SPELT COOKIES

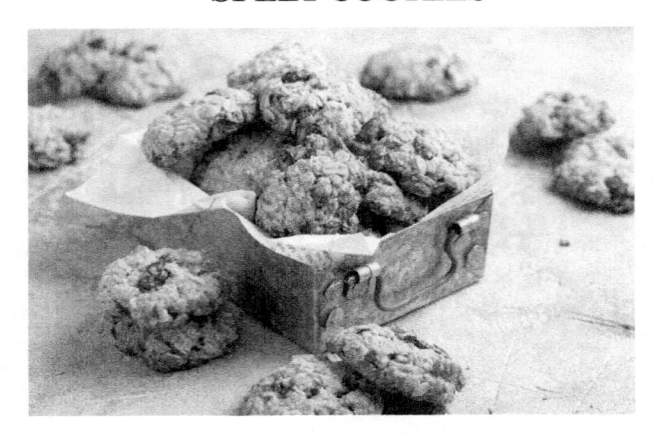

Cooking Time: 45 Minutes
Serving Size: 24 Cookies

Ingredients

- 1-1/2 cups of Spelt Flour
- 1-1/2 of pitted Dates
- 1-1/2 rolled Spelt Flakes
- 1 cup of Raisins
- 2/3 cup of prepared *Applesauce (see recipe on page 129)*
- 1/3 cup of Grapeseed Oil
- 1/3 cup of Agave Syrup
- 1/2 teaspoon of Pure Sea Salt
- 2 tablespoons of Sparkling Spring Water

Cooking Instructions

1. Add Dates, Spelt Flour, and Pure Sea Salt in a food processor and blend them well.
2. Put prepared mixture into a bowl, add *Applesauce*, Spelt Flakes, Raisins, Sparkling Spring Water, Agave Syrup, and Grapeseed Oil. Mix them until well combined.
3. Preheat your oven to 350°F. Take a cookie sheet and cover it with parchment paper.

4. Take a spoonful of the dough in your hand, form a ball, and put it on the cookie sheet. Flatten it with a fork or your fingers.
5. Bake cookies for about 20 minutes.
6. Serve and enjoy your Spelt Cookies!

COCONUT TAHINI COOKIES

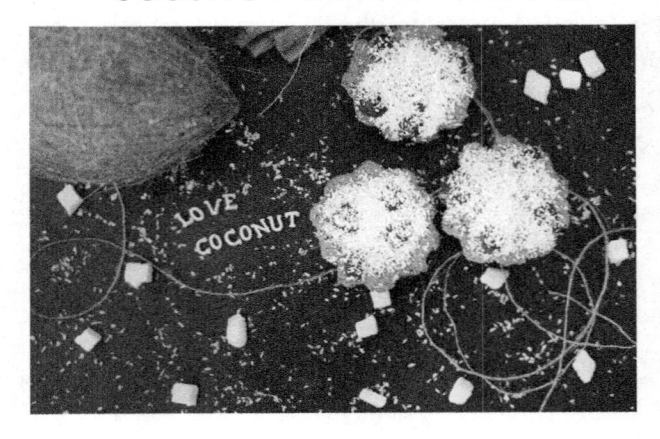

Cooking Time: 30 Minutes
Serving Size: 8 Cookies

Ingredients

- 1 cup of Unsweetened Coconut Flakes
- 1/4 cup of Agave Syrup
- 1 tablespoon of *Homemade Tahini Butter (see recipe on page 111)*
- 2 tablespoons of Coconut Oil
- Pinch of Pure Sea Salt

Cooking Instructions

1. Put all ingredients in a blender or a food processor. Pulse 5 times and then blend for 20 seconds until well mixed.
2. Put prepared mixture into cupcake liners with a spoon.
3. Freeze it for about 15–20 minutes to set coconut oil and firm up the cookies.
4. Serve and enjoy your Coconut Tahini Cookies!

Useful Tips

You can add dried fruits or nuts from *Dr. Sebi's Food List (check it on page 22).*

TEFF TAHINI COOKIES

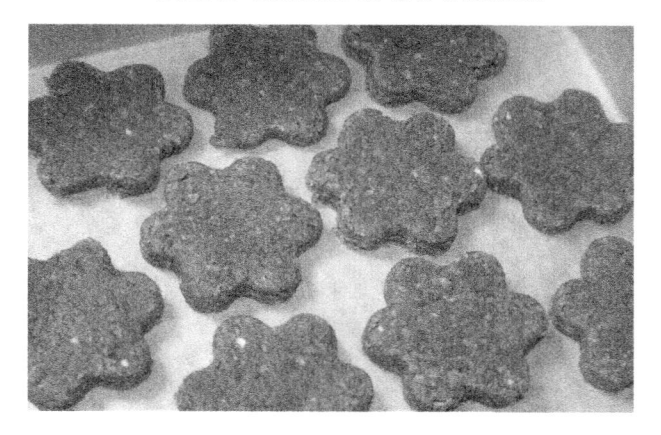

Cooking Time: 40 Minutes
Serving Size: 15–18 Cookies

Ingredients
- 1-1/4 cups of Teff Flour
- 2/3 cup of Agave Syrup
- 2/3 cup of *Homemade Tahini Butter (see recipe on page 111)*
- 1/4 cup of Grapeseed Oil
- 1/4 teaspoon of Pure Sea Salt

Cooking Instructions
1. Preheat your oven to 350°F.
2. Put Agave Syrup, *Homemade Tahini Butter,* and Grapeseed Oil in a bowl and mix them. Add Teff Flour and Pure Sea Salt to the mixture and blend well.
3. Take a cookie sheet and cover it with parchment paper.
4. Take a spoonful of the dough in your hand, form a ball, and put it on the cookie sheet half an inch apart. Gently flatten it with a fork or fingers.
5. Repeat the step 4 until all the dough is used. Bake cookies for about 10–12 minutes.
6. Serve and enjoy your Teff Tahini Cookies!

STRAWBERRY BANANA ICE CREAM

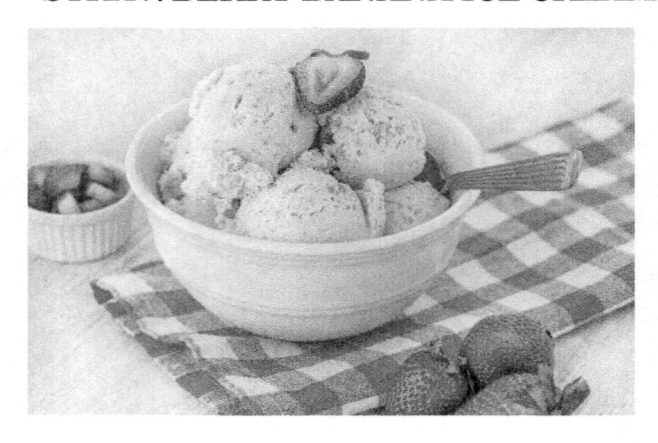

Cooking Time: 4 Hours
Serving Size: 5 Servings

Ingredients

- 1 cup of Strawberry*
- 5 quartered Baby Bananas*
- 1/2 chopped Avocado
- 1 tablespoon of Agave Syrup
- 1/4 cup of *Homemade Walnut Milk (see recipe on page 107)***

Cooking Instructions

1. Put all above-mentioned ingredients into a blender and mix them well.
2. Taste cooked mixture. If you think it is too thick, add extra *Homemade Walnut Milk***. If you want it sweeter, add extra Agave Syrup.
3. Place the mixture in a container with a lid. Allow it to freeze for at least 5–6 hours.
4. Serve and enjoy your homemade Strawberry Banana Ice Cream!

Useful Tips

* If you don't have fresh bananas or berries, you can use frozen ones.

Add any fruits you like from *Dr. Sebi's Food List (check it on page 22),* but be sure to use avocado every time. The fat, which includes Avocado, helps to achieve a creamier consistency.

** If you don't have *Homemade Walnut Milk*, you can substitute it with *Homemade Hempseed Milk (see recipe on page 114).*

SMOOTHIES

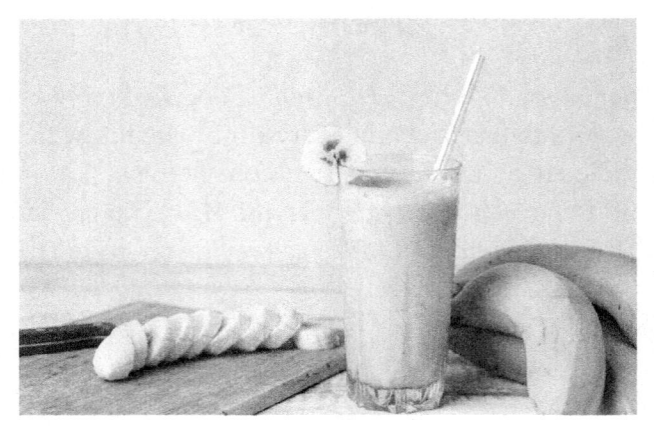

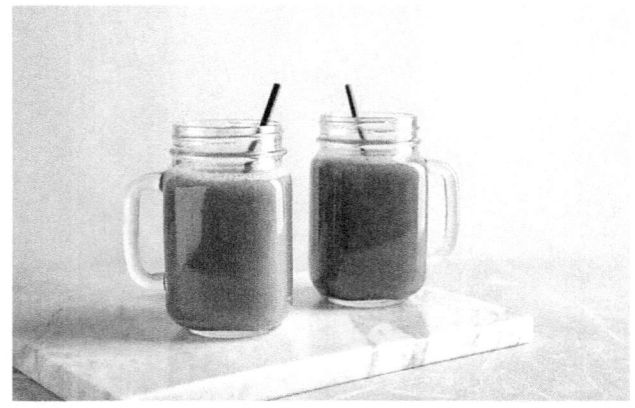

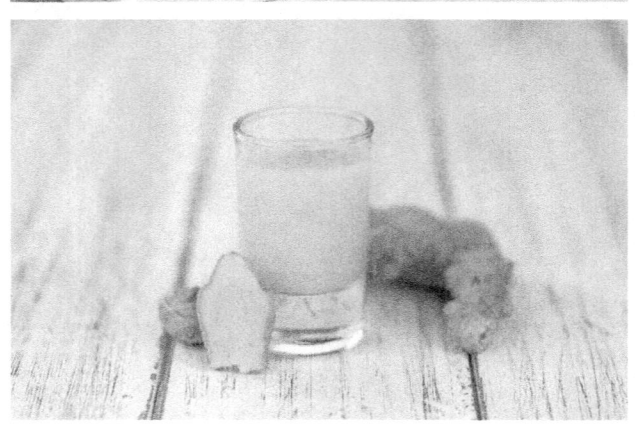

SOURSOP SMOOTHIE

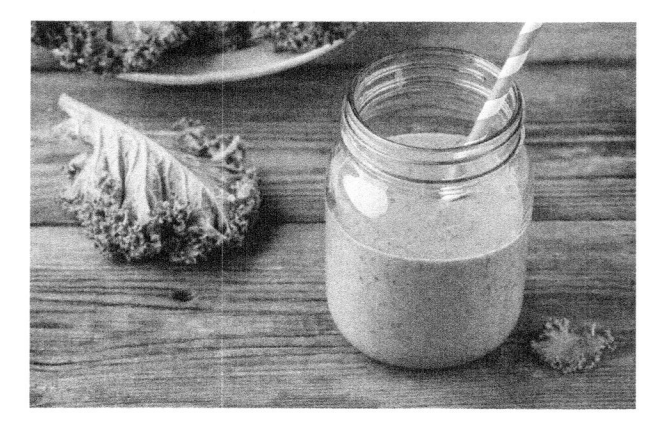

Cooking Time: 5 Minutes
Serving Size: 2 Servings

Ingredients
- 3 quartered frozen Burro Bananas*
- 1-1/2 cups of *Homemade Coconut Milk (see recipe on page 110)*
- 1/4 cup of Walnuts
- 1 teaspoon of Sea Moss Gel
- 1 teaspoon of Ground Ginger
- 1 teaspoon of Soursop Leaf Powder
- 1 handful of Kale

Cooking Instructions
1. Prepare and put all ingredients in a blender or a food processor.
2. Blend it well until you reach a smooth consistency.
3. Serve and enjoy your Soursop Smoothie!

Useful Tips
* If you don't have frozen Bananas, you can use fresh ones.

HEALTHY SMOOTHIE

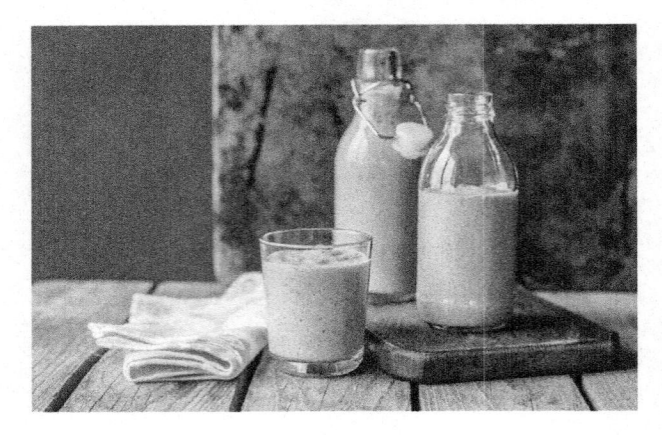

Cooking Time: 10 Minutes
Serving Size: 2 Servings

Ingredients

- 1 seeded Cucumber
- 1/4 of an Avocado
- 1/4 of a Pear
- 1/4 of an Apple
- 1 Burro Banana*
- 1 teaspoon Bromide Plus Powder
- 1 cup of Lettuce
- juice from 1 Key Lime
- 1 cup of Spring Water

Cooking Instructions

1. Put the Lettuce and Spring Water in a blender. Blend them well until you get a smooth liquid.
2. Peel the Cucumber, chop it, and put it in the blender. Blend all together.
3. Add pieces of Banana, Apple, and Pear in the blender. Blend it repeatedly until all chunks are not visible.

4. Add Avocado with Bromide Plus Powder in the blender. Continue blending until a creamy consistency is reached.
5. Serve and enjoy your Healthy Smoothie!

Useful Tips

* If you don't have the Burro Banana, you can add 2 Baby Bananas instead.

LIMEADE

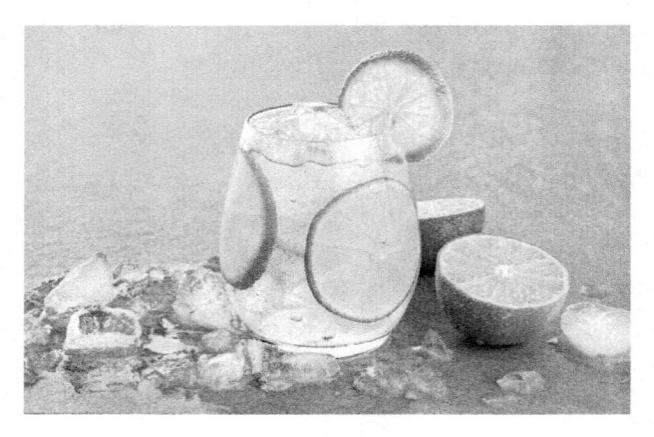

Cooking Time: 15 Minutes
Serving Size: 2 Servings

Ingredients
- 1/4 cup of Lime Juice
- 1/4 cup of Agave Syrup
- 2 cups of Spring Water

Cooking Instructions
1. Pour all ingredients in a blender or a food processor.
2. Blend it well for 10–20 seconds.
3. Allow to cool in a refrigerator for 10–15 minutes or add some ice.
4. Serve and enjoy your Limeade!

CUCUMBER-GINGER WATER

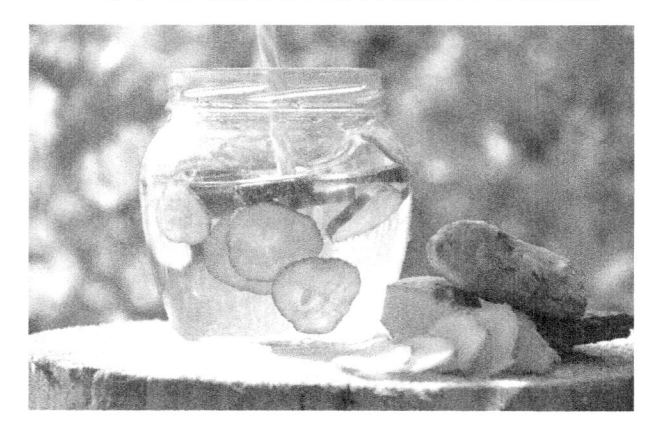

Cooking Time: 5 Minutes + night for infusion
Serving Size: 2 Servings

Ingredients
- 1 sliced Cucumber
- 1 smashed thumb of Ginger Root
- 2 cups of Spring Water

Cooking Instructions
1. Prepare and put all ingredients in a jar with a lid.
2. Let the water infuse overnight. Store it in the refrigerator.
3. Serve and enjoy your Cucumber-Ginger Water throughout the day!

STRAWBERRY MILKSHAKE

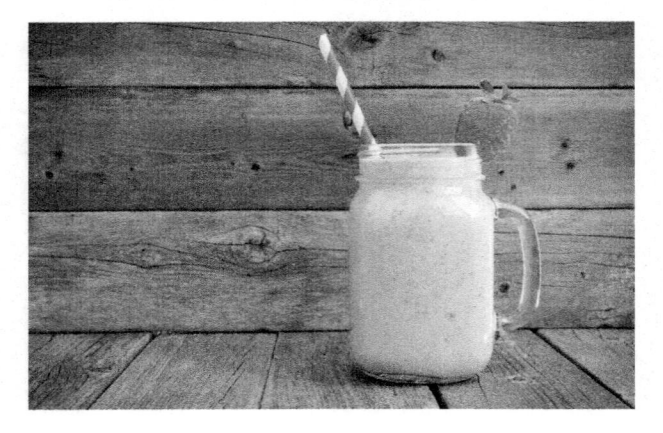

Cooking Time: 5 Minutes
Serving Size: 2 Servings

Ingredients
- 2 cups of *Homemade Hempseed Milk (see recipe on page 114)**
- 1 cup of frozen Strawberries**
- Agave Syrup, to taste

Cooking Instructions
1. Prepare and put all ingredients in a blender or a food processor.
2. Blend it well until you reach a smooth consistency.
3. Serve and enjoy your Strawberry Milkshake!

Useful Tips
* If you don't have *Homemade Hempseed Milk,* you can add *Homemade Walnut Milk (see recipe on page 107)* instead.
** If you don't have frozen Strawberries, you can use fresh ones.

CACTUS SMOOTHIE

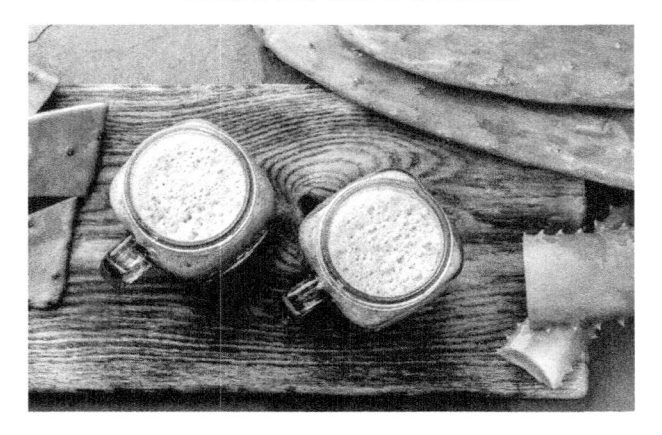

Cooking Time: 10 Minutes
Serving Size: 2 Servings

Ingredients
- 1 medium Cactus
- 2 cups of *Homemade Coconut Milk (see on page 110)**
- 2 frozen** Baby Bananas or 1 Burro Banana
- 1/2 cup of Walnuts
- 1 Date
- 2 teaspoons of Hemp Seeds

Cooking Instructions
1. Take the Cactus, remove all pricks, wash it, and cut into medium pieces.
2. Put all ingredients in a blender or a food processor.
3. Blend it well until you reach a smooth consistency.
4. Serve and enjoy your Cactus Smoothie!

Useful Tips
* If you don't have *Homemade Coconut Milk,* you can add *Homemade Walnut Milk (see on page 107)* or *Hempseed Milk (see on page 114)* instead.
** If you don't have frozen Bananas, you can use fresh ones.

PRICKLY PEAR JUICE

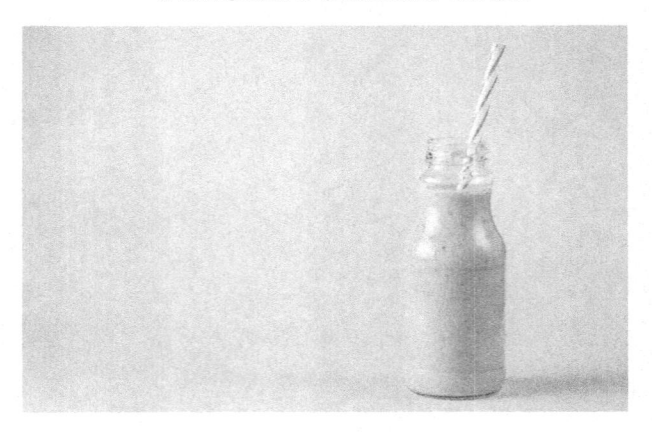

Cooking Time: 10 Minutes
Serving Size: 2 Servings

Ingredients
- 6 Prickly Pears
- 1/3 cup of Lime Juice
- 1/3 cup of Agave
- 1-1/2 cups of Spring Water*

Cooking Instructions
1. Take Prickly Pear, cut off the ends, slice off the skin, and put in a blender. Do the same with the other pears.
2. Add Lime Juice with Agave to the blender and blend well for 30–40 seconds.
3. Strain the prepared mixture through a nut milk bag or cheesecloth and pour it back into the blender.
4. Pour Spring Water* in and blend it repeatedly.
5. Serve and enjoy your Prickly Pear Juice!

Useful Tips
* If you want a cold drink, add a tray of ice cubes instead.

GINGER TEA

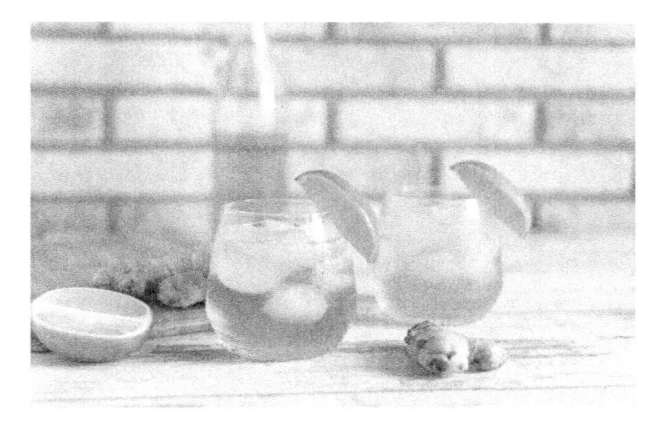

Cooking Time: 10 Minutes
Serving Size: 4 Servings

Ingredients
- 1 thumb of Ginger Root
- 4 cups of Spring Water
- 2 springs of Dill Weed
- 2 tablespoons of Lime Juice
- 1 pinch of Cayenne Powder
- Agave, to taste

Cooking Instructions
1. Pour Spring Water into a medium pot and bring to a boil.
2. Peel a Ginger Root and chop it.
3. Add Dill Weed and chopped Ginger Root to boiling water. Allow to cook for 5 minutes.
4. Strain cooked tea into a bowl.
5. Add Lime Juice and stir it.
6. Add Agave and Cayenne Powder, to taste.
7. Serve and enjoy your Ginger Tea!

BANANA MILKSHAKE

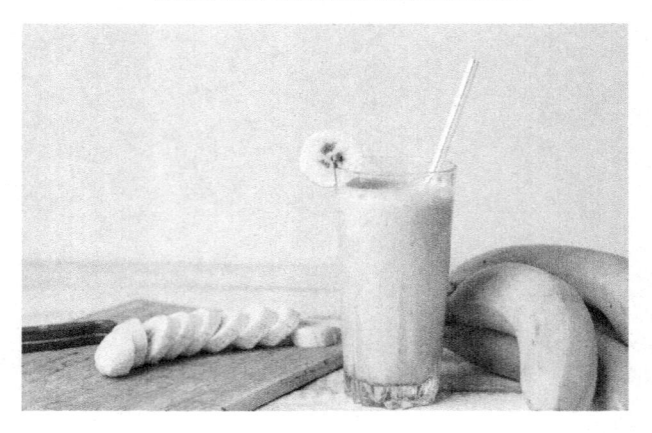

Cooking Time: 5 Minutes
Serving Size: 1 Serving

Ingredients
- 6 frozen* Baby Bananas or 3 Burro Bananas
- 1/4 cup of *Homemade Hempseed Milk (see recipe on page 114)****
- 1/8 teaspoon of Cloves
- 1 tablespoon of Agave Syrup

Cooking Instructions
1. Prepare and put all ingredients in a blender or a food processor.
2. Blend it well until you reach a smooth consistency. If it is too thick, add extra *Homemade Hempseed Milk.***
3. Serve and enjoy your Banana Milkshake!

Useful Tips
* If you don't have frozen Bananas, you can use fresh ones.
** If you don't have *Homemade Hempseed Milk,* you can add *Homemade Walnut Milk (see recipe on page 107),* or *Homemade Coconut Milk (see recipe on page 110)* instead.

STRAWBERRY LIMEADE

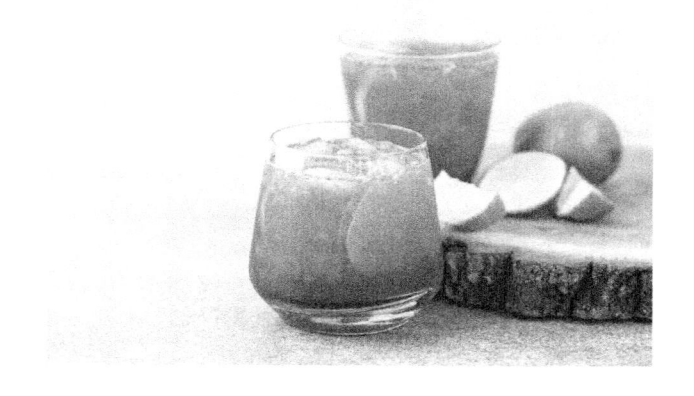

Cooking Time: 5 Minutes
Serving Size: 2 Servings

Ingredients
- 1/2 cup of Strawberries
- 1/4 cup of Lime Juice
- 1/4 cup of Agave Syrup
- 1 cup of Spring Water
- 6–8 Ice Cubes

Cooking Instructions
1. Wash Strawberries, cut off the leaves, and cut berries in half.
2. Put all ingredients in a blender or a food processor.
3. Blend it well for 10–20 seconds or until you reach a smooth consistency.
4. Serve and enjoy your Strawberry Limeade!

SOURSOP TEA

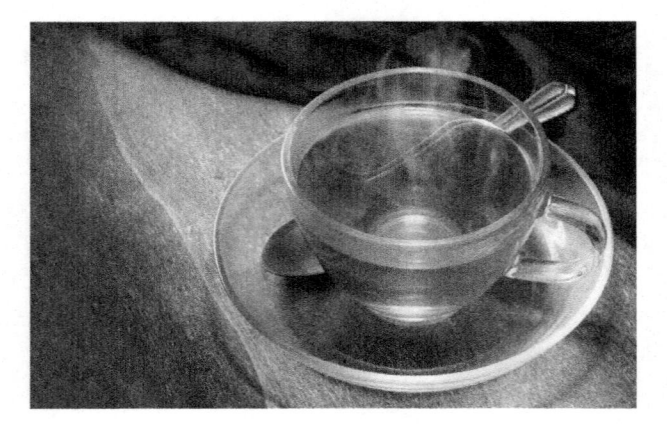

Cooking Time: 15 Minutes
Serving Size: 2 Servings

Ingredients
- 1–2 Soursop Leaves
- 1–1-1/2 cups of Spring Water

Cooking Instructions
1. Rinse Soursop Leaves before using them.
2. Boil Spring Water.
3. Add Leaves to boiling Spring Water.
4. Allow to steep for 15 minutes.
5. Serve and enjoy your Soursop Tea!

Useful Tips
Drink up to two cups of this Soursop Tea during the day to reach the best results.

GINGER SHOT

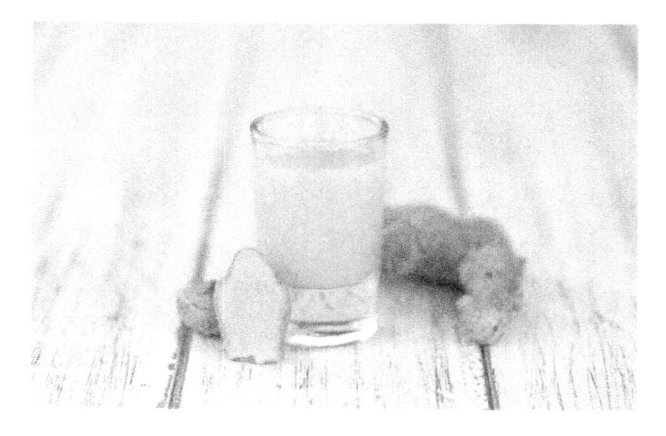

Cooking Time: 10 Minutes
Serving Size: 1 Serving

Ingredients

- 1/4 cup of Ginger Root
- 1 small Apple
- 1–2 cups of Spring Water

Cooking Instructions

1. Peel the Ginger Root and chop it.
2. Peel the Apple and cut it into pieces.
3. Add chopped Ginger Root and cut Apple in a blender.
4. Pour Spring Water into a blender.
5. Blend it well for 30–60 seconds.
6. Strain the mixture through a nut milk bag or a cheesecloth.
7. Serve and enjoy your Ginger Shot!

GREEN SMOOTHIE

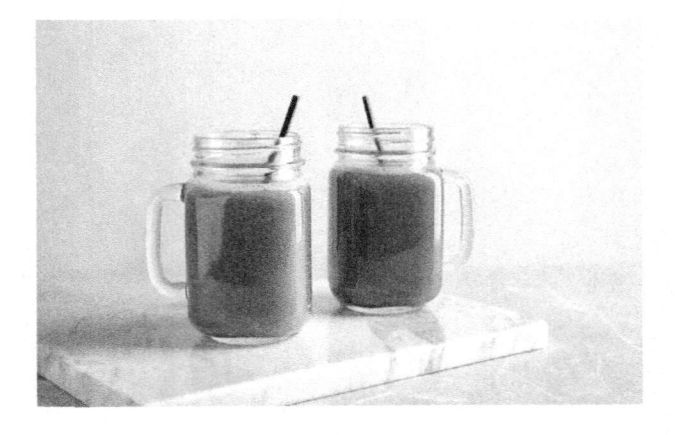

Cooking Time: 5 Minutes
Serving Size: 2 Servings

Ingredients
- 1 cup of *Homemade Coconut Milk (see recipe on page 110)*
- 2 frozen** Burro Bananas***
- 2 cups of Arugula
- 2 teaspoons of Sea Moss Gel

Cooking Instructions
1. Prepare and put all ingredients in a blender or a food processor.
2. Blend it well until you reach a smooth consistency.
3. Serve and enjoy your Green Smoothie!

Useful Tips
* If you don't have *Homemade Coconut Milk*, you can add *Homemade Walnut Milk (see recipe on page 107) or Homemade Hempseed Milk (see recipe on page 114)* instead.
** If you don't have frozen Bananas, you can use fresh ones.
*** If you don't have Burro Bananas, add 4 Baby Bananas instead.

PEACH STRAWBERRY SMOOTHIE

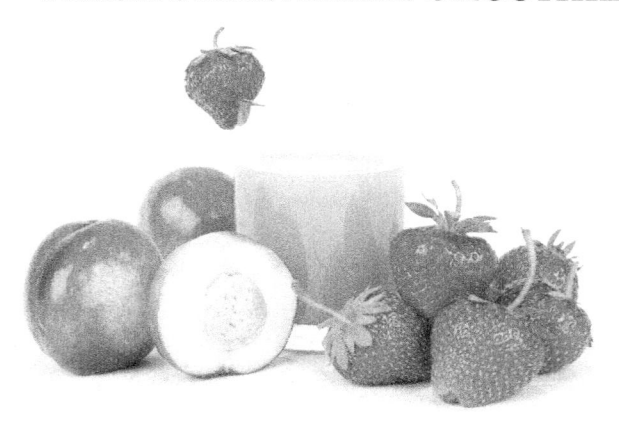

Cooking Time: 5 Minutes
Serving Size: 2 Servings

Ingredients

- 2–3 cups of *Homemade Coconut Milk (see on page 110)**
- 1 cup of frozen** Peaches
- 1 cup of frozen** Strawberries
- 2 teaspoons of Hemp Seeds
- 2 teaspoons of Sea Moss Gel
- 2 Dates

Cooking Instructions

1. Prepare and put all ingredients in a blender or a food processor.
2. Blend it well until you reach a smooth consistency.
3. Serve and enjoy your Peach Strawberry Smoothie!

Useful Tips

* If you don't have *Homemade Coconut Milk*, you can add *Homemade Walnut Milk (see on page 107)* or *Homemade Hempseed Milk (see on page 114)* instead.
** If you don't have frozen Bananas, you can use fresh ones.

CONCLUSION

Congratulations!

Now you have learned 77 simple, Dr. Sebi alkaline diet recipes. That means you can surprise yourself, your family, and your friends with new, delicious dishes, snacks, salads, desserts, or smoothies.

Not only will you be eating tasty meals, you will also be helping yourself and your family to feel better and improve overall health just by eating approved Dr. Sebi food. How great is that?

Now there is just one thing for you to do: Take action!

I know, you have most likely been in this position before. Maybe you have already tried other diets in the past, but you just can't find a suitable nutritional plan for you.

This time will be different. I promise!

Take care of yourself and live a long, healthy life!

Printed in Great Britain
by Amazon